DRINK YOUR OWN WATER

A Treatise on Urine Therapy

Tony Scazzero

Llumina
Press

Disclaimer

This book is not a replacement for medical diagnosis, treatment, or advice. The information in this booklet is based on the author's research and experience. For those who want to heal themselves, it is an overview to a free, alternative medicine. If you begin this treatment for a specific ailment, try it at your own risk and please accept responsibility for the results. Healing through this method may cause the body to detoxify, which can cause unpleasant reactions. When the body is immunized by its own medicine, true healing takes place. Further study and investigation is recommended.

Tony Scazzero

www.drinkyourownwater.com

Requests for permission to make copies of any part of this work should be mailed to Permissions Department, Llumina Press, 7101 W. Commercial Blvd., Ste. 4E, Tamarac, FL 33319

ISBN: 978-1-60594-855-3 (PB)
       978-1-60594-875-1 (EB)

Printed in the United States of America by Llumina Press

Library of Congress Control Number: 2012901383

To God, the true parent of all mankind, who gave us the capability to heal ourselves.

CONTENTS

PREFACE

Lady Dr. Kim

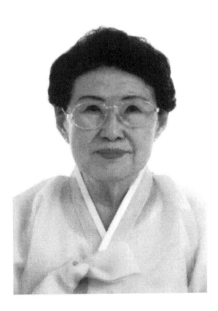

When I traveled to the spirit world to learn how to help my brothers and sisters maintain their health, the Heavenly Father gave me a cup of yellow liquid that was my own urine. He said it works to cure all kinds of sicknesses, both internally and externally. Tons of antibiotics are not as effective as this medicine. It doesn't sound good, but it is the Heavenly Father's gift to us. People are spending billions of dollars on costly medical care, but you have the cure right inside your body.

INTRODUCTION

*D*rink *Your Own Water* is another way of saying urine therapy so that the readers can begin to learn to adjust their concepts of urine from something unpleasant to something that sounds natural. Urine therapy has not been able to go mainstream for two major reasons. One is that most people cannot overcome their initial reaction of displeasure and revulsion. Two, because the medical establishment is against alternative therapies especially if there is no money in it. The intention of this book is to help get the message out that urine therapy is a better alternative than the current medical system for many diseases. Ironically, many people are spending huge amounts of money on substandard treatment when most can be treated by this free, simple home remedy. Even more staggering is that many people experience serious pain and even lost of life because they do know about the alternatives that are considered "unproven." Regrettably, large numbers of people die prematurely from diseases that can be easily controlled by means of urine therapy.

The majority of environmental threats to our health are the result of an unprecedented explosion in the manufacture, use, and release of radiation and chemicals. It is estimated that over a hundred thousand chemicals are now produced in commercial volumes. Trillions of tons of toxic substances are released into the air, water, soil, and ecosystems each year. These carcinogens cause not only sicknesses, but birth defects, developmental, and reproductive problems. Is it any coincidence that diseases are on the increase as pollutants, radiation, and toxins are increasing every year?

Today, the dangerous list of toxins in our air, food, and water is disturbing. Most chemicals in our environment didn't exist one hundred years ago, so their long-term effect on our health is still unknown. Our houses are loaded with chemicals as toxins can be found in our personal care products, our cleaning products, and in our food. The average American diet consists of fast foods and processed foods loaded with salt and sugar. The body's immune systems are being overburdened by the constant intake of toxic chemicals. There are over twenty heavy metals (arsenic, lead, mercury, cadmium . . .) around us that accumulate in the soft tissues of the body. These can cause serious neurological damage even before birth. Phthalates (plasticizers) and fire retardants are in almost everything we use. More than eighty thousand chemicals are utilized every day, yet most of them have never been fully accessed for toxic impacts on human health and the environment. Combine this with the enormous radioactive fallout from nuclear weapons testing and active power plants, and the result is problematical to say the least

The medical communities have been busy dealing with the vast increase in health problems from these man-made actions. On one hand, modern medicine has done a great job extending and saving people's lives. On the other, it has not been able to overcome many dreadful diseases such as cancer, polio, asthma, AIDS, lupus, and diabetes. Medical researchers have produced significant accomplishments in the last one hundred years, yet new maladies like superbugs, swine flu, and H1N1 are on the increase and some old ones, e.g., whooping cough, measles, and tuberculosis are hard to eradicate. Conventional medicine should be truthful about their inability to handle diseases efficiently and effectively.

There are many natural, integrative therapies available to help reduce casualties from both communicative and noncommunicative diseases. Society has not given the naturalistic way the funding or acceptance that traditional medicine has received. Physicians, with sophisticated equipment, perform dozens of tests, yet malpractice, misdiagnosis, and wrong drug prescriptions continue unabated. In the hospital, a sick person is monitored around the clock and treated with painkillers and antibiotics for their symptoms. These methods actually weaken the immune system and weaken the body's own disease-fighting mechanisms. They interfere with the production of antibodies while creating addictions to those drugs. This traditional approach compounds the initial problems and does not address the cause. Meanwhile, medical costs are skyrocketing, as are the medical mistakes. Doctors oftentimes perform risky procedures and prescribe toxic drugs. Despite increased medical technology, modern medical science has yet to come up with a cure for even the common cold.

In the meantime, every year, almost eight million people worldwide die from cancer. The lifetime probability of developing cancer is one in two for men and one in three for women. Even as research and treatment has increased dramatically and funding has soared, the number of men and women diagnosed with cancer continues to rise. The government has spent billions of dollars for medical treatments that has no definitive success in curing patients. There have been massive resources thrown at these medical problems, but drugs and surgery remain the foremost response for most of them. Furthermore, drug companies along with the government (FDA) have suppressed natural remedies. It is time to stop the madness and start thinking for ourselves how to maintain a healthy lifestyle. It is more than inconvenient to be stricken with a disease and have no cure. Sooner or later, individuals have to learn how to take responsibility to prevent sickness and to heal themselves.

CHAPTER 1

THE STATISTICS

The sheer magnitude of the number of people with diseases is overwhelming and increasing every year. By conservative estimates there are over fifty thousand diseases worldwide that affect us. To say we are have a health epidemic is an understatement. Nobody is untouched by some form of sickness. Many of their causes and cures are still unknown. Here are just some figures of illnesses (in the United States alone) that does not include the undiagnosed!

⅄	Allergies	50,000,000
⅄	Arthritis	21,000,000
⅄	Asthma	20,000,000
⅄	AIDS	1,000,000
⅄	Alzheimer's	5,100,000
⅄	Anemia	3,000,000
⅄	Diabetes	26,000,000
⅄	Digestive Diseases	70,000,000
⅄	Cancers	12,000,000
⅄	Cardiovascular disease	80,000,000
⅄	Cholera	5,000,000
⅄	Chronic fatigue syndrome	1,000,000
⅄	Crohn's disease	1,400,000
⅄	Fibromyalgia	5,000,000
⅄	Heart disease	26,800,000
⅄	Hepatitis A,B,C	5,300,000

⋏	Influenza	50,000,000
⋏	Lupus	1,500,000
⋏	Mold illnesses	5,000,000
⋏	Pneumonia	3,000,000
⋏	Sexually transmitted diseases	65,000,000

Around the world, diseases like tuberculosis, yellow fever, smallpox, malaria, cholera, measles, and meningitis have wiped out millions of people. Today, communicable diseases are on the rise while new ones are appearing as bacteria, viruses, fungi, and protozoa and have become more drug resistant. Outbreaks of polio, Avian influenza, West Nile Virus, severe acute respiratory syndrome, MRSA, and infectious diseases present a global challenge. Pandemics from natural disasters, radiation, bioterrorism along with food and water poisoning are issues that will not go away. In short, the threat of disease is always close by. A large percentage of the world lacks access to health care. The ones that have, put their lives in jeopardy by submitting to risky treatments. What is the cause of these problems and more importantly what is the solution?

CHAPTER 2

HUMAN EXPOSURES TO ENVIRONMENTAL POLLUTANTS

Whether it is workplace exposures, household exposures or naturally occurring exposures, people care about what in their environment may cause disease. Over the past century, technology has introduced a huge number of chemical substances into the environment. These chemicals benefit society, but their harm and toxicity far outweigh their benefits. The production, trade and use of chemicals have been increasing geometrically globally. The result of this growth has been accompanied by a broad range of negative impacts on human health. There has been a wide range of consequences depending on the length and intensity of the exposure, genetic makeup and the strength of the person's immune system. Toxic chemicals impact health with genetic mutations, cancers, birth defects, neurological problems along with dysfunctions of the endocrine, reproductive and immune systems.

The dominant sources of air pollution today are industrial facilities (led by coal-fired power plants, metal smelters, pulp and paper mills, petroleum refineries, and chemical factories), mobile sources (diesel trucks, heavy-duty vehicles, cars, trains, planes, and boats), agriculture and residential burning of fossil fuels, and wood. Industrial facilities spew billions of tons of pollutants into the air and water annually, including known or suspected carcinogens such as styrene, benzene and formaldehyde. There are almost one billion cars on our planet earth exhausting sulfur dioxide, nitrogen oxides, particulate matter and carbon dioxide as well as thousands of other hazardous air pollutants. Exposure to air pollution can cause a host of afflictions. The result of decreased lung function and respiratory infections can lead to asthma attacks, bronchitis, heart attacks, strokes, cancer and premature death.

Persistent Organic Pollutants (POPs) are the leading group of chemicals that are the most toxic and can cause cancer and other adverse health effects. The twelve most persistent organic pollutants are aldrin, endrin, chlordane, DDT, dieldrin, dioxins and furans, heptachlors, hexachlorobenzene, mirex, PCBs and toxaphene. POPs are persistent in the environment and can travel vast distances via air and water. Although non-government organizations like the International POPs Elimination Network and the Pesticide Action Network are working to stem their proliferation, more and more chemicals are being developed every year.

The risks of toxic chemicals in our food, water and air have been established, yet the link between pollution and health is a relatively new phenomenon. The Environmental Working Group compared the ingredient list of over fourteen thousand personal care products to the lists of potential chemical hazards compiled by the EPA, FDA, the International Agency for Research on Cancer, the European Chemicals Bureau and thirty other scientific and regulatory institutions around the world. The end result was that a large number of chemicals found in household products, including cosmetics and personal care products, instigate harmful effects. Their manufacture and use cause a large number of chemicals to get into air, food and drinking water. A child born today faces increased odds of developing at least one or more of the following ailments: asthma, autism, attention deficit hyperactivity disorder, diabetes, obesity, childhood and pubertal cancers, abnormal genitalia development and infertility. Even breast and prostate cancers, Parkinson's, and Alzheimer's have joined the list of disorders that have been linked to prenatal exposure to toxic chemicals. Billions of dollars a year in medical bills can be attributed to the health effects caused by exposure to chemicals.

Despite prodigious amounts of money spent on research, the United States does not have a viable means of keeping its three hundred million citizens safe from the untold chemical hazards in the things that we use day in and day out. Large amount of carcinogens are in our work and living environment, e.g., chlorine in most municipal water supplies, insecticides, pesticides, food additives and fire-retardant materials that jeopardize our safety. Consequently, chemicals that interfere with the body's reproductive, developmental and behavioral systems are freely used on everything from plastics, soaps and toys to food wrappers, clothing and carpeting.

Many of these chemicals are hormonal disruptors. They throw off the body's hormone system in various ways and cause lab animals to exhibit disorders and diseases, that coincidentally are on the rise in humans. These diseases include cancers of the breast, testicles and brain; lower sperm count; early puberty; endometriosis and other defects of the female reproductive system; obesity; attention deficit disorder; diabetes; asthma; and autism. These chemicals are now found at low levels in countless applications, in everything from personal care products and cooking pans to electronics, furniture, clothing, building materials and children's toys. The chemical industry insists that everyday exposures are inconsequential because the amounts are too minuscule to matter.

The Environmental Protection Agency's Office of Chemical Safety and Pollution Prevention has been able to order tests on only a few hundred chemicals and take action on only a handful. The Toxic Substances and Control Act of

1976, the Pollution Prevention Act and the Safe Chemicals Act are basically ineffective because they discourage chemical companies from sharing hazard and exposure information. They are weak because they do not really protect the public. As a result, everyone, everywhere now carries a dizzying array of chemical contaminants—the by-products of modern industry and innovation. These toxic substances accumulate in our fat, bones, blood, and organs and are responsible for dreadful health problems including cancer, birth deformities, neurological impairments, and disruption of the hormonal system. As the earth rotates every day, the most persistent chemicals are carried across oceans and continents by water and air. They're fat soluble and they biomagnify, increasing in concentration as they move up the food chain. When they reach humans, their combinations magnify, causing a chemical body burden that many immune systems cannot handle.

In the United States, the chemical influence includes more than eighty thousand industrial substances registered for commercial purposes with the EPA. The Center for Disease Control tracks dozens of pesticides and chemical compounds we encounter in daily life. There are hundreds of other chemicals for which the means to screen for their presence has not yet been developed. There are over 150 chemicals in gasoline alone, including benzene, which is a known human carcinogen. Every day in the United States alone, over ninety million barrels a day of petroleum and over nineteen million barrels of gasoline are used up. The vast majorities of these do not biodegrade or break down in the environment. The government has to create new agencies just to handle this demand on society.

The CDC has shown that phthalates exposure is widespread, and according to the FDA, at least five different phthalates are present in cosmetics and personal care products. Levels of PBDEs in human fat, blood and breast milk in North

America—the largest user of flame retardants—are ten to one hundred times higher than those reported for Europe and Asia. Pollutants that persist in the environment, such as DDT, PCBs dioxin, lead and mercury, hitch themselves to the body's fatty tissues. Bisphenol A (BPA) leaches from containers into our food and beverages, and everyone is exposed within the dose range that causes devastating problems in animals. Even low-dose Bisphenol A results in functional and structural changes in the prostate, breasts, testes and mammary glands. The lists of diseases and adverse health conditions now plausibly linked to Bisphenol A by animal and cell research is large with the possibility that BPA may eventually alter human development.

Mounting evidence suggests that tiny amounts of certain chemicals, both natural and synthetic, can wreak havoc with hormones that shape our bodies and behavior over a lifetime. Endocrine disruptors causes reduction in male fertility, declines in the number of males born, abnormalities in male reproductive organs, female reproductive diseases including early puberty, and increases in cancers of the breast, ovaries and prostate. Another hazardous substance that has been found in the blood of everybody in the United States is perfluorooctanoic acid (PFOA). PFOA is used by Du Pont to make the nonstick substance known as Teflon. The EPA's scientific advisory panel advised classifying PFOA as a likely human carcinogen— causing cancer, birth defects and other reproductive harm. Almost every industry uses these fluoropolymer applications including aerospace, automotive, construction, chemical processing, electronics, semiconductors and textiles.

Another similar chemical pollutant is perfluorooctanesulfonic acid (PFOS) used for firefighting foams, hydraulic fluids, alkaline cleaners, floor polishes, photographic film, denture cleaners, shampoos and insecticides. Environmental regulators are particularly alarmed because scientists are finding PFOA in the blood of people worldwide, and it takes years for the chemical to leave the body. Research data show they are persistent, bioaccumulative, and toxic in the environment. After forty years of manufacture and distribution, many have been phased out, yet their detection is still found in food, wildlife and humans.

According to the Environmental Protection Agency, indoor air is more polluted than outside air, due largely to all the emissions from furnishings, paints, foams, insulators, fire retardants, veneers, flooring as well as dust, dander, and sometimes cigarette smoke. Synthetic wall-to-wall carpet is loaded with chemicals. Chemical-filled household cleaning products are linked to cancer, immune system disorders, liver damage, reproductive problems in men, behavioral problems in children and many other common health issues. Heavy metals such as mercury, cadmium, arsenic, chromium, and lead compounds are regularly emitted into our environment and consumer products. They affect and disrupt many brain functions since they have a high affinity for fat, which makes up 90 percent of our brain.

Water is another source of toxicity today. Our tap water is treated with chlorine to kill microscopic organisms and fluoride to strengthen teeth. Chlorine is universally used to chemically disinfect tap water. Yet chlorine is a toxic chemical that has been linked to an increase incidence of colon and bladder cancer. There is also a connection between fluoride and osteoporosis, increased blood pressure and an increase of problems with the thyroid gland. Fluoride is a known toxin and is linked to problems with the kidneys, the central nervous system and the skeletal system. It is also linked to cancers and lower IQs. Run-off from industrial toxins and wastes make it through water treatment facilities in trace amounts and into our tap water. A recent study showed that forty-one million

Americans drink water contaminated with antidepressants, hormones, heart medications and other prescription and over-the-counter medications that have made it through the water treatment system. The water in our showers and bathtubs has potentially greater toxicity because we absorb more water through our skin when bathing than when drinking.

Moreover, the electromagnetic fields (EMF) around us from cell phones, power lines, computer screens, microwaves, military radar, transformers and electrical appliances have been linked to serious health problems. Can EMFs cause brain tumors, leukemia, birth defects, miscarriages, chronic fatigue, headaches, asthma, nausea, forgetfulness, cancer and other health problems? Studies have shown a consistent pattern of the affects of chronic exposure to EMFs. The proliferation of cell phones and other wireless devices have led to human populations being surrounded by EMFs of increasing intensity. EMF is being recognized as a critical missing link in understanding the escalating levels for so many diseases today. It is estimated that we are exposed to a trillion times more EMF than our grandparents were. The EPA advice of prudent avoidance suggests there are a wide range of health effects due to EMF exposure. The National Institute of Occupational Safety and Health has been researching electric and magnetic fields to protect workers from possible health risks. Studies, both public and private, are continuing; however, political and economic influence from utility, military, and computer lobbyists may sway the outcomes of these studies.

By and large, chemical regulations benefit the industry at the expense of the public. Environmental regulators largely rely on companies that profit from industrial chemicals to sound alarms about their safety, but it doesn't usually happen until a serious problem develops. The studies of the health effects of multiple chemicals are in its infancy because of the lack of scientific understanding of chemical interactions in humans and due to their complexity. Fundamentally, the cumulative risk assessment of many chemicals is still unexplored. It is hard enough to understand the effects of one chemical, let alone thousands, because it takes many years of use and study to understand the outcomes.

Medical experts have no idea whether carcinogenic chemicals are twenty or a hundred times more likely to cause cancer or whether their effects are immediate or latent. At any rate, the United States and Europe are seeing rising rates of infertility among males and females, increasing rates of endocrine-related malformations and neurological disorders that scientists attribute to the effects of toxic chemicals. The U.S. Centers for Disease Control tested for 171 toxic chemicals in 2010 and discovered their presence in the bodies of Americans of all ages.

The National Toxicology Program has an interagency program within the Department of Health and Human Services that works to safeguard public health by identifying the effects of everyday chemicals. The National Toxicology Program brings together three agencies: the National Institute of Environmental Health Sciences of the National Institute of Health (NIEHS/NIH), the National Institute for Occupational Safety and Health of the Centers for Disease Control and Prevention (NIOSH/CDC), and the National Center of Toxicological Research of the Food and Drug Administration (NCTR/FDA). These are just a few of the government programs that have been established with billions of dollars to track chemically induced health problems. Their job is to research diseases that are linked to environmental exposures, for example, asthma, autism, breast cancer, and Parkinson's disease. They have to choose at what level of exposure these toxins have the potential of becoming hazardous to humans.

The primary method to test the toxicity of chemicals is by the use of chemical disposition on animals. This science of toxicokinetics studies the absorption of the chemical and how it spreads through the animal tissue. It also explains how they transform the animal's metabolism and its effects on the animal urine and feces. Toxicokinetics examines the changes of the concentration of the chemical over time in the blood or other tissues. Then this data on laboratory animals is applied to humans through mathematical modeling. Another more direct way to determine chemical effects in humans is biomonitoring studies using mass spectrometers for the detection of trace quantities of contaminants or toxins. In general, lengthy studies have been made to understand their potential effects on humans based on their effects in animals. The question of how to reverse toxic contaminations has not been fully addressed yet. The National Institute for Occupational Safety and Health (NIOSH) has their own list of 132 potential occupational carcinogens. The International Agency for Research on Cancer has evaluated and categorized over nine hundred chemicals. The U.S. Environmental Protection Agency (EPA) maintains the Integrated Risk Information Systems, an electronic database that contains human health effects from exposures of 550 substances in the environment. The Department if Health and Human Services 2011 12th Report on Carcinogens looks at 254 toxins and is 499 pages long. The Toxic Release Inventory (TRI) analysis is an annual report that displays EPA's analysis and interpretation of the most recent TRI data. It includes a dizzying array of toxic chemical disposal or other releases to the environment. It also includes trends in toxic chemicals managed by TRI facilities, and analyses of certain chemicals of interest, industry sectors, parent companies and geographic areas. These exhaustive government researches are very informative; however, they are very weak on prevention or treatment. The scientific explanations of their carcinogenicity, properties, use and exposure would challenge the most meticulous scientist. Just the partial list of these known carcinogens is hard to comprehend, and it is just the tip of the iceberg.

1. Acrylamide
2. Acrylonitrile
3. Adriamycin
4. Aflatoxins
5. Alcoholic Beverage Consumption
6. 2-Aminoanthraquinone
7. o-Aminoazotoluene
8. 4-Aminobiphenyl
9. 1-Amino-2,4-dibromoanthraquinone
10. 1-Amino-2-methylanthraquinone
11. Amitrole
12. o-Anisidine and Its Hydrochloride
13. Aristolochic Acids
14. Arsenic and Inorganic Arsenic Compounds
15. Asbestos
16. Azacitidine
17. Azathioprine
18. Basic Red 9 Monohydrochloride
19. Benzene
20. Benzidine and Dyes Metabolized to Benzidine
A. Benzidine
B. Dyes Metabolized to Benzidine (Benzidine Dye Class)
21. Benzotrichloride
22. Beryllium and Beryllium Compounds
23. 2,2-Bis(bromomethyl)-1,3-propanediol (Technical Grade)
24. Bis(chloromethyl) Ether and Technical-Grade Chloromethyl Methyl Ether
25. Bromodichloromethane
26. 1,3-Butadiene

27. 1,4-Butanediol Dimethanesulfonate
28. Butylated Hydroxyanisole
29. Cadmium and Cadmium Compounds
30. Captafol
31. Carbon Tetrachloride
32. Ceramic Fibers (Respirable Size)
33. Chlorambucil
34. Chloramphenicol
35. Chlorendic Acid
36. Chlorinated Paraffins (C12, 60% Chlorine)
37. Chloroform
38. 3-Chloro-2-methylpropene
39. 4-Chloro-o-phenylenediamine
40. Chloroprene
41. p-Chloro-o-toluidine and Its Hydrochloride
42. Chromium Hexavalent Compounds
43. Cisplatin
44. Coal Tars and Coal-Tar Pitches
45. Cobalt Sulfate
46. CobaltTungsten Carbide: Powders and Hard Metals
47. Coke-Oven Emissions
48. p-Cresidine
49. Cupferron
50. Cyclophosphamide
51. Cyclosporin A
52. Dacarbazine
53. Danthron
54. 2,4-Diaminoanisole Sulfate
55. 2,4-Diaminotoluene
56. Diazoaminobenzene
57. 1,2-Dibromo-3-chloropropane
58. 1,2-Dibromoethane
59. 2,3-Dibromo-1-propanol

60. 1,4-Dichlorobenzene
61. 3,3'-Dichlorobenzidine and Its Dihydrochloride
62. Dichlorodiphenyltrichloroethane
63. 1,2-Dichloroethane
64. Dichloromethane
65. 1,3-Dichloropropene (Technical Grade)
66. Diepoxybutane
67. Diesel Exhaust Particulates
68. Di(2-ethylhexyl) Phthalate
69. Diethylstilbestrol
70. Diethyl Sulfate
71. Diglycidyl Resorcinol Ether
72. 3,3'-Dimethoxybenzidine and Dyes Metabolized to 3,3'-Dimethoxybenzidine
    A. 3,3'-Dimethoxybenzidine
    B. Dyes Metabolized to 3,3'-Dimethoxybenzidine (3,3'-Dimethoxybenzidine Dye Class)
73. 4-Dimethylaminoazobenzene
74. 3,3'-Dimethylbenzidine and Dyes Metabolized to 3,3'-Dimethylbenzidine
    A. 3,3'-Dimethylbenzidine
    B. Dyes Metabolized to 3,3'-Dimethylbenzidine (3,3'-Dimethylbenzidine Dye Class)
75. Dimethylcarbamoyl Chloride
76. 1,1-Dimethylhydrazine
77. Dimethyl Sulfate
78. Dimethylvinyl Chloride
79. 1,4-Dioxane
80. Disperse Blue
81. Epichlorohydrin
82. Erionite
83. Estrogens, Steroidal
84. Ethylene Oxide

85. Ethylene Thiourea
86. Ethyl Methanesulfonate
87. Formaldehyde
88. Furan
89. Certain Glass Wool Fibers (Inhalable)
90. Glycidol
91. Hepatitis B Virus
92. Hepatitis C Virus
93. Heterocyclic Amines (Selected)
    A. 2-Amino-3,4-dimethylimidazo[*4,5-f*]quinoline
    B. 2-Amino-3,8-dimethylimidazo[*4,5-f*]quinoxaline
    C. 2-Amino-3-methylimidazo[*4,5-f*]quinoline
    D. 2-Amino-1-methyl-6-phenylimidazo[*4,5-b*]pyridine
94. Hexachlorobenzene
95. Hexachloroethane
96. Hexamethylphosphoramide
97. Human Papillomaviruses: Some Genital-Mucosal Types
98. Hydrazine and Hydrazine Sulfate
99. Hydrazobenzene
100. Ionizing Radiation
    A. X-Radiation and Gamma Radiation
    B. Neutrons
    C. Radon
    D. Thorium Dioxide
101. Iron Dextran Complex
102. Isoprene
103. Kepone
104. Lead and Lead Compounds
105. Lindane, Hexachlorocyclohexane (Technical Grade), and Other Hexachlorocyclohexane Isomers
106. Melphalan
107. Methoxsalen with Ultraviolet A Therapy
108. 2-Methylaziridine

109. 4,4'-Methylenebis(2-chloroaniline)
110. 4,4'-Methylenebis(N,N-dimethyl)benzenamine
111. 4,4'-Methylenedianiline and Its Dihydrochloride
112. Methyleugenol
113. Methyl Methanesulfonate
114. Metronidazole
115. Michlers Ketone
116. Mineral Oils: Untreated and Mildly Treated
117. Mirex
118. Mustard Gas
119. Naphthalene
120. 2-Naphthylamine
121. Nickel Compounds and Metallic Nickel
    A. Nickel Compounds
    B. Metallic Nickel
122. Nitrilotriacetic Acid
123. o-Nitroanisole
124. Nitroarenes (Selected)
    A. 1,6-Dinitropyrene
    B. 1,8-Dinitropyrene
    C. 6-Nitrochrysene
    D. 1-Nitropyrene
    E. 4-Nitropyrene
125. Nitrobenzene
126. Nitrofen
127. Nitrogen Mustard Hydrochloride
128. Nitromethane
129. 2-Nitropropane
130. rN-Nitrosamines: 15 Listings
    A. *N*-Methyl-N'-Nitro-*N*-Nitrosoguanidine
    B. *N*-Nitrosodi-n-butylamine
    C. *N*-Nitrosodiethanolamine
    D. *N*-Nitrosodiethylamine

E. *N*-Nitrosodimethylamine

F. *N*-Nitrosodi-n-propylamine

G. *N*-Nitroso-*N*-ethylurea

H. 4-(*N*-Nitrosomethylamino)-1-(3-pyridyl)-1-butanone

I. *N*-Nitroso-*N*-methylurea

J. *N*-Nitrosomethylvinylamine

K. *N*-Nitrosomorpholine

L. *N*-Nitrosonornicotine

M. *N*-Nitrosopiperidine

N. *N*-Nitrosopyrrolidine

O. *N*-Nitrososarcosine

131. Nitrosourea Chemotherapeutic Agents

A. Bis(chloroethyl) Nitrosourea

B. 1-(2-Chloroethyl)-3-cyclohexyl-1-nitrosourea

C. 1-(2-Chloroethyl)-3-(4-methylcyclohexyl)-1-nitrosourea

D. Chlorozotocin

E. Streptozotocin

132. o-Nitrotoluene

133. Norethisterone

134. Ochratoxin A

135. 4,4'-Oxydianiline

136. Oxymetholone

137. Phenacetin and Analgesic Mixtures Containing Phenacetin

A. Phenacetin

B. Analgesic Mixtures Containing Phenacetin

138. Phenazopyridine Hydrochloride

139. Phenolphthalein

140. Phenoxybenzamine Hydrochloride

141. Phenytoin and Phenytoin Sodium

142. Polybrominated Biphenyls

143. Polychlorinated Biphenyls

144. Polycyclic Aromatic Hydrocarbons: 15 Listings

A. Benz[*a*]anthracene

B. Benzo[*b*]fluoranthene

C. Benzo[*j*]fluoranthene

D. Benzo[*k*]fluoranthene

E. Benzo[*a*]pyrene

F. Dibenz[*a,h*]acridine

G. Dibenz[*a,j*]acridine

H. Dibenz[*a,h*]anthracene

I. 7H-Dibenzo[*c,g*]carbazole

J. Dibenzo[*a,e*]pyrene

K. Dibenzo[*a,h*]pyrene

L. Dibenzo[*a,i*]pyrene

M. Dibenzo[*a,l*]pyrene

N. Indeno[*1,2,3-cd*]pyrene

O. 5-Methylchrysene

145. Procarbazine and Its Hydrochloride

146. Progesterone

147. 1,3-Propane Sultone

148. β-Propiolactone

149. Propylene Oxide

150. Propylthiouracil

151. Reserpine

152. Riddelliine

153. Safrole

154. Selenium Sulfide

155. Silica, Crystalline (Respirable Size)

156. Soots

157. Strong Inorganic Acid Mists Containing Sulfuric Acid

158. Styrene

159. Styrene-7,8-oxide

160. Sulfallate

161. Tamoxifen

162. 2,3,7,8-Tetrachlorodibenzo-p-dioxin

163. Tetrachloroethylene
164. Tetrafluoroethylene
165. Tetranitromethane
166. Thioacetamide
167. 4,4'-Thiodianiline
168. Thiotepa
169. Thiourea
170. Tobacco-Related Exposures
    A. Tobacco Smoking
    B. Environmental Tobacco Smoke
    C. Smokeless Tobacco
171. Toluene Diisocyanates
172. o-Toluidine and Its Hydrochloride
173. Toxaphene
174. Trichloroethylene
175. 2,4,6-Trichlorophenol
176. 1,2,3-Trichloropropane
177. Tris(2,3-dibromopropyl) Phosphate
178. Ultraviolet Radiation Related Exposures
    A. Solar Radiation
    B. Exposure to Sunlamps or Sunbeds
    C. Broad-Spectrum UVR
    D. UVA
    E. UVB
    F. UVC
179. Urethane
180. 4-Vinyl-1-cyclohexene Diepoxide
181. Vinyl Halides (Selected)
    A. Vinyl Bromide
    B. Vinyl Chloride
    C. Vinyl Fluoride
182. Wood Dust

CHAPTER 3

THE FOOD IS NOT SAFE

Much of the food we are eating is not safe. Each year, according to the Centers for Disease Control, more than 48 million Americans are made sick by the food they eat. Of these, some 128,000 require hospital care and 3,000 die from "food-borne illness." Processed foods, genetically modified foods and irradiated foods are damaging to our health. The Food and Drug Administration has found that much of the food harvested contain pesticide residues, chemical contaminates and extraneous materials. These pesticides are not only burdensome to the immune systems of humans, but to animals and plants as well.

Every year, hundreds of pesticides, many of them known to be detrimental to the nervous and reproductive system, are used on farms to "protect the public" from pests. Over 50 percent of grocery foods contain pesticide residues. These fruit and vegetables are covered with residues known to be carcinogenic. The pesticides and chemicals we eat get deposited inside body fat. Researchers have found high concentrations of DDT, PCBs dieldrin, heptachlor, dioxin and other agricultural chemicals in human blood samples taken across the country and the globe! Pesticides are designed to disrupt the hormonal and neurological systems of insects, but they also affect children's physical and mental growth. Yet, their exact impact on public health has not been established.

We consume foods that have been depleted of essential natural healing nutrients. These nutrients have been replaced by synthetic chemical additives. These additives in our processed foods interact with the thousands of chemicals absorbed from our air, water and consumer products, further undermining our immune system. Then we become susceptible to illnesses that medical practitioners treat with synthetic chemical drug compounds that increases our toxicity even more. Our diets from birth to death are now shaped by processed food corporations that promote synthetics as harmless and even superior to natural foods. Processed foods are less digestible and more inflammatory than natural foods. Chemists have been working with food-processing companies to create artificial sweeteners, taste enhancing additives such as MSG and partially hydrogenated vegetable shortening that are linked to cardiovascular diseases. In short, the over consumption of refined sugar and white flour along with food additives are having a deleterious effect on the general public. As a result, many health problems can be attributed to nutritional deficiencies found in the modern diet. There is an illusion of food safety because of the existence of the Food and Drug Administration and the Environmental Protection Agency. Consumer protection laws along with legal standards like the Pure Food and Drug Act are meant to prevent food-related health problems. Yet nutrition is declining while diseases are growing.

Some of the facts are particularly disturbing for parents.Food additives and artificial preservatives account for much of the hyperactivity and behavioral problems in children. Meanwhile, dietary deficiencies of vitamin and minerals are hindering school performance with refined carbohydrates being a factor in juvenile diabetes. The Centers for Disease Control found over one hundred toxic substances in the bodies of the average adult in America, with children carrying an even higher level of synthetic chemicals. The epidemics of obesity and cancer point to a dietary weakness common in the modern Western diet.

Food-borne diseases are more prevalent with contaminated food, causing hundreds of disease outbreaks every year. The number and prevalence of bacterial diseases has grown dramatically since the industrialization of animal farms. Some of which include salmonella, campylobacter, E.coli, listeria and vibrio cholerae. Regularly occurring E. coli and salmonella outbreaks sicken millions of people worldwide every year. A host of chronic ailments, including reactive arthritis, Reiter's syndrome, Miller-Fisher syndrome and ulcers have now been linked to bacterial infections often caused by contaminated foods. Exacerbating this growing epidemic is the fact that human antibiotics have been losing their effectiveness. Partly because over 80 percent of the soy and 38 percent of the corn planted in the United States are genetically engineered.

The spread of toxins continues to affect both environmental and public health. Carcinogens are not only found in the bodies of the vast majority of human beings but in the bodies of wild and domestic animals and in most major rivers and groundwater. Many of these chemicals combine in a toxic gathering that is harmful to fish and the broader freshwater ecosystem. Since the late 1970s, studies have found more than 139 different pesticide residues in groundwater in the United States. American farmers use close to one billion pounds of pesticides a year. Nearly every pesticide has been detected in the air, rain, snow or fog across the nation at different times of the year. Many pesticides contaminate our water long after their use was discontinued. Despite the ban on DDT in 1972, it still finds its way into our soil, vegetables, water and bloodstream today.

Most of the health problems today are caused by dietary abuses. Factory-made foods have made chemicals additives part of our diet. Some additives appear to be safe while others may injure us in large amounts. Sugar and salt are ubiquitous in most of our meals. Sugar substitutes found in pudding, chewing gum, nondairy creamers, instant coffee mixes, tea mixes and gelatin desserts may increase cancer in humans. Processed foods are manipulated with food additives, sweeteners, flavorings, coloring agents, preservatives, bleaching agents, emulsifiers, texturizers, humectants, acids, alkalis and buffers to prolong shelf life. Such foods provide loads of calories but little health benefit. Fast food and fried foods fatten our bodies and shorten our lives. We are overfed with processed foods yet in reality undernourished. In addition, genetically engineered foods produce their own pesticide so they introduce new allergens, toxins, disruptive chemicals and unknown protein combinations when we ingest them.

You have to be a chemist or a biologist to comprehend most of the added ingredients in supermarket foods. Most of which should be avoided:

- ✓ Corn syrup
- ✓ Dextrose (corn sugar, glucose)
- ✓ Fructose
- ✓ Hydrogenated starch hydrolysate
- ✓ Invert sugar
- ✓ Lactitol
- ✓ Maltitol
- ✓ Mannitol
- ✓ Polydextrose
- ✓ Salatrim
- ✓ Salt
- ✓ Sorbitol
- ✓ Sugar
- ✓ Tagatose
- ✓ Xylitol
- ✓ Artificial colorings: blue 1, citrus red 2, red 40
- ✓ Brominated vegetable oil (BVO)

- ✓ Butylated hydroxytoluene (BHT)
- ✓ Diacetyl
- ✓ Heptyl Paraben
- ✓ Stevia/Rebiana
- ✓ Natural flavoring: annatto
- ✓ Caffeine
- ✓ Carmine/Cochineal
- ✓ Casein
- ✓ Guarana
- ✓ Gum arabic (acacia)
- ✓ Gum Tragacanth
- ✓ Hydrolyzed vegetable protein (HVP)
- ✓ Lactose
- ✓ Mycoprotein/quorn
- ✓ Quinine
- ✓ Sodium Benzoate
- ✓ Sodium Bisulfite
- ✓ Sodium Caseinate
- ✓ Sulfites
- ✓ Sulfur dioxide
- ✓ Acesulfame-k
- ✓ Artifical colorings: blue 2, green 3, orange B, red 3, yellow 5, yellow 6
- ✓ Aspartame (NutraSweet)
- ✓ Butylated hydroxyanisole (BHA)
- ✓ Caramel coloring
- ✓ Cyclamate (not legal in United States)
- ✓ Olestra (Olean)
- ✓ Partially hydrogenated vegetable oil (trans fat)
- ✓ Potassium bromate
- ✓ Propyl gallate
- ✓ Saccharin

Moreover, many of the common chemicals listed below are suspected or known carcinogens, hormone disruptors, or contaminants. Their affects are not inspiring.

Acetone

Also known as dimethyl ketone, 2-propanone, beta-ketopropane. Inhalation of moderate to high amounts, even for a short time, results in entry of acetone into bloodstream where it is carried to all other organs. A known nose, throat, lung, and eye irritant, it also causes headaches, confusion, increased pulse rate, bad effects on blood, nausea, vomiting and unconsciousness, coma. It shortens the menstrual cycle in women. Effects of long-term exposure include kidney, liver, and nerve damage, increased birth defects, metabolic changes, and coma. It is found in nail polish remover.

Acetaldehyde

Found in many nail care products. Known to cause cancers in humans and experimental animals.

Acrylamide/Polyacrylamide

Acrylamide is produced naturally in some foods when cooked at high temperatures. Manufactured for use in polyacrylamide gels, it is sometimes used as a treatment for drinking water and/or wastewater. Acrylamide causes cancer in animals and, when ingested in large doses, nerve damage in humans. Smoking is a major acrylamide producer as is frying, deep-frying, or extended microwaving.

Alcohol

Implicated in oral cancer. Found in mouthwash, astringent, toothpaste, cleansers.

Alkyl-phenol Ethoxylates

May reduce sperm count. Found in shampoo and bubble bath.

Alpha Hydroxy Acid

Destroys skin cells and leaves skin more susceptible to damage from the environment and skin cancer. Actually ends up aging skin. Found in antiaging facial creams and lotions.

Aluminum

Heavy concentrations may be linked to Alzheimer's dementia. Aluminum is in many antiperspirants and prevalent in water supplies. Processed foods contain dietary aluminum. Sodium aluminum phosphate appears in pickles, cheese, and baking soda.

Ammonium Glycolate

A photosensitizer with potential to increase risk of sunburn and skin cancer by intensifying UV exposures in deep skin layers. This sensitizer can instigate immune system response that includes itching, burning, scaling, hives, and blistering of skin. It is also a penetration enhancer, which alters the skins' structure, allowing other chemicals to penetrate deeper into the skin, thus increasing the amounts of other chemicals that reach the bloodstream. Found in body products.

Ammonium Persulfate

Found in hair color and bleaching kit sensitizer—can instigate immune system response that can include itching, burning, scaling, hives, and blistering of skin, lung sensitizer; can instigate immune system response that can include asthma attacks or other problems with the lungs and airways.

Aspartame

Genetically modified synthetic sugar substitute. People report dizziness, headaches, and even seizures. Scientists believe it can alter behavior due to altered brain function. Long-term effects of this genetically modified organism on human health has not been studied or tested. Found as a sweetener in foods and some body products, such as shaving gel.

Benzalkonium Chloride, Cetrimonium Chloride, and Lauryl Dimonium Hydrolyzed Collagen

Found in hair treatment products. Both are toxic and allergenic.

Benzene

Inhalation of high levels can cause headaches, rapid heart rate, tremors, confusion, unconsciousness, and death. Hodgkin's lymphomas result from inhalation. Used in detergents, drugs, pesticides, and adhesives.

Benzoic Acid

Inhalation affects nervous system and is moderately toxic by ingestion. Severe eye and skin irritant. Used as a food preservative and in pharmaceuticals and cosmetics.

Benzoic/Benzyl/Benzene

Contains carcinogens, endocrine disruptor; may cause birth defects. Found in shower gels, shampoos, bubble bath.

Benzoyl Peroxide

Found in acne treatments, bar soaps, facial cleansers, and food additives. Highly toxic/ irritant.

Bisphenol A or BPA

Toxic plastic chemical used as a can lining in brands of some infant formulas. Also found in water bottles, this chemical is used to produce polycarbonate and epoxy plastics. For babies, check food container labels and beware of polycarbonate plastic baby bottles. Chemical reactions can occur when plastic is heated.

BHA and BHT

Banned in other countries, these two preservatives are considered carcinogenic, but they remain in U.S. manufactured foods that contain oil as they retard rancidity. Found in many foods and body products.

Bronopol

May break down into formaldehyde; may form carcinogenic nitrosamines. Found in body products.

Butylparaben

Potential breast cancer risk and endocrine disruptor, raising concern for impaired fertility or development, increased risk for certain cancers; causes itching, burning and blistering of skin. Found in body products.

Carboxymethylcellulose

Causes cancer in animals. Used in cosmetics; inhalation could cause chemical pneumonitis.

Coal Tar Dyes (includes D and C blue 1, green 3, yellow 5, yellow 6, red 33, etc.)

Even though their carcinogenicity has recently been proven, the 1938 act includes a specific exemption for them. Severe allergic reactions, asthma attacks, headaches, nausea, fatigue, lack of concentration, nervousness, increased risk of Hodgkin's disease, non-Hodgkin's lymphoma, and multiple myeloma. Found in bubble bath, hair dye, dandruff shampoo, toothpaste, and foods.

Cocamidopropyl Betaine

May contain harmful impurities or form toxic breakdown products that cause itching, burning, and blistering of skin. Synthesized from coconuts, this chemical is found in body products and may be labeled natural or organic.

Coumarin

Formerly the active ingredient in rat poison. A carcinogenic ingredient used in the manufacturing of deodorants, shampoos, skin fresheners, and perfumes.

D and C Yellow 11

Found in: lip gloss, polish remover, nail polish, bath oil/salts/soak, body spray, mositurizer, lipstick, styling gel/lotion, bar soap, after sun products, cologne, and nail treatment. Color is safe for external use only; found in ingested products. Color not approved for use around eyes. Found in eye products

DEA: Diethanolamine

A chemical used as a wetting or thickening agent in shampoos, soaps, hairsprays and sunscreens; blocks absorption of the nutrient choline, which is essential to brain development in a fetus.

Diacetyl

An additive that tastes like butter but causes a serious lung condition called bronchiolitis obliterans, or "popcorn workers' lung." Found in foods, especially microwave popcorn.

Dibutyl phthalate (DBP)

A chemical used to keep nail polish from chipping, it has been connected to cancer in lab animals as well as long-term fertility issues in newborn boys. Banned in Europe but still in use in the United States. Found in nail polish.

Dimethicone

A silicone emollient, which coats the skin not allowing toxins out. May promote tumors and accumulate in the liver and lymph nodes. Found in lotions and creams.

Dioforms

Damage and weaken tooth enamel, allowing more staining and discoloration to take place. Found in tooth-whitening products.

Disodium EDTA

Harmful if swallowed or inhaled; causes irritation to skin, eyes, and respiratory tract. Found in cosmetics.

Diazolidinyl Urea

Found in facial cleansers, shampoos, and conditioners. Linked to neurotoxicity and immunotoxicity

DMDM Hydantoin

Contains formaldehyde , an ingredient linked to cancer and developmental and reproductive toxicity. Allergenic, can be an irritant to eyes skin and lungs. Common in manicure/pedicure products and hair treatment packages.

Ethyl Acrylate

Found in some mascaras; suspected as a cause of cancer in humans based on studies of human populations or laboratory animals.

Elastin

Suffocates skin by not allowing moisture in or out. Found in facial creams and body lotions.

Fluoride

May contain lead, mercury, cadmium, and arsenic. Accumulates in body and contributes to bone disease. Carcinogenic. Found in toothpastes.

Formaldehyde

Suspected carcinogen and neurotoxin, it may be fatal if swallowed, absorbed through skin, or inhaled. Can cause spasms, edema, chemical pneumonitis, and is extremely destructive to tissue of the mucous membrane. This chemical is found in many nail care products. Known to cause cancers in humans and experimental animals. Found in baby shampoo, bubble bath, deodorants, perfume, cologne, hair dye, mouthwash, toothpaste, hair spray, nail polish.

Fragrances (Synthetic)

Some perfumes/fragrances contain hundreds of chemicals. Some, such as methylene chloride, are carcinogenic. Some cause brain damage or are neurotoxins. Avoid unless you can be sure they are not carcinogenic.

Glycolic Acid

Penetration enhancer, which alters skin structure, allowing other chemicals to penetrate deeper into the skin, increasing the amounts of other chemicals that reach the bloodstream, skin, or sense organs. As a sensitizer, it can instigate immune system response that can include itching, burning, scaling, hives, and blistering of skin. Toxicant, neurotoxin, kidney toxicant, gastrointestinal, or liver toxicant. Found in creams, lotions, cosmetics.

GMO/Genetically Modified Organism

Plants, animals, or foods that have been genetically modified, genetically engineered or BT/biotechnology modified. Genetic engineering enables scientists to create plants, animals and microorganisms by manipulating genes in a way that does not occur naturally. Minimal testing shows that animals fed GMO feed refuse to eat it. When force-fed with the feed (corn, soy, tomatoes, etc.), the animals developed stomach lesions and malformations of organs. GMO food is not labeled as such in the United States. Almost all other countries have banned the use of GMO in food and body products due to insufficient testing.

Hydroabietyl Alcohol

Found in styling gel/lotions. Unsafe for use in cosmetics according to the fragrance industry's International Fragrance Association.

High-Fructose Corn Syrup/HFCS

High fructose consumption has been fingered as a causative factor in heart disease. It raises blood levels of cholesterol and triglycerides. It makes blood cells more prone to clotting, and it may also accelerate the aging process.

Hydrogenated/Partially Hydrogenated Oils

Hydrogenated oils contain high levels of trans fats. A trans fat is an otherwise normal fatty acid that has been radically changed by high heat. Trans fats are poison, just like arsenic. Partially hydrogenated oils will not only kill you in the long term by producing diseases like multiple sclerosis and allergies that lead to arthritis, but in the meantime, they will also make you fat!

Hydroquinone

A severely toxic and very powerful chemical. Banned in the United Kingdom but still used in the United States. Found in skin lightening products and hair dyes, this chemical alters the skins natural structure, inhibiting the production of melanin. Without natural protection, the skin is more susceptible to skin cancer. Prolonged use of hydroquinone will thicken collagen fibers, damaging the connective tissues. The result is rough blotchy skin, leaving it with a spotty caviar appearance.

Hydroxyethyl Cellulose

Used in cosmetics. Inhalation could cause chemical pneumonitis.

Imidazolidinyl Urea

This allergenic chemical finds its way into deodorants, shampoos, hand cream, and some mascaras.

Isobutylparaben

Potential breast cancer risk. Itching, burning, and blistering of skin. Found in body products.

Isopropanol/Isopropyl Alcohol

Moderately toxic chemical causing flushing, pulse rate decrease, blood pressure lowering, anesthesia, narcosis, headache, dizziness, mental depression, drowsiness, hallucinations, distorted perceptions, respiratory depression, nausea, vomiting, and coma. Used to clean/disinfect skin and lower temperatures. Found in some body products.

Kojic Acid

A chemical that inhibits melanin production. Used in skin lightening products, it damages the skin and makes it more susceptible to cancer.

Lacquer

Can cause eyelashes to fall out. Found in mascara.

Lanolin

While lanolin itself is skin beneficial, it may contain carcinogenic pesticides such as DDT, lindane, dieldrin, and other neurotoxins. Can cause rashes. Found in body products.

Lye

Can dry and damage skin. Found in bars of soap.

Magnesium Stearate/Stearic Acid

May contain phosphatidylcholine, which collapses cell membranes and selectively kills T-cells, which breaks down the immune system. An execeptant that is used to bind medicinal tablets and make them smooth. It is also used in pharmaceuticals, foods, talcum powder, ammunition, and as a drying agent in paints.

MEA: Cocamide DEA, Lauramide DEA, Linoleamide DEA, Oleamide DEA

NDEA (N-nitrosodiethanolamine) forms when DEA reacts with nitrosating agents or the actual addition of nitrite as a preservative. As there is no way to determine if NDEA has been formed, it is imperative to avoid all products containing DEA as it is a known carcinogen. Often used in cosmetics to adjust the pH, and used with many fatty acids to convert acid to salt (stearate), this then becomes the base for a cleanser.

Methylisothiazolinone or MIT

Causes neurological damage. Found in shampoo.

Methyl Methacrylate

May cause fingers and nails to inflame. Found in nail polish.

Methylparaben

Potential breast cancer risk and endocrine disruptor, raising concern for impaired fertility or development of fetus, and increases risk for certain cancers; causes itching, burning and blistering of skin. A close cousin of benzoic acid; poisonous and moderately toxic, it is found in body products.

Mineral Oil

A derivative of petroleum, this additive clogs pores, locks in toxins, suffocates and dries skin, and inhibits your skin's natural oil production, further increasing dehydration. Causes testicular tumors in the fetus, deposits accumulate in the lymph nodes, and prevents absorption of vitamin A from the intestines. Found in blush, baby oil, lotions, foundation, and creams.

Monosodium Glutamate/MSG

MSG is an excitotoxin, which causes nerve damage and allergic reactions. Found in hundreds of foods, often under other names.

MTBE

Gasoline additive. Known as a "likely" human carcinogenic.

Neotame

A reformulated aspartame that will require smaller amounts than aspartame to achieve the same sweetness. Neotame, like aspartame, contains aspartic acid, phenylalanine, and a methyl esther. Animal studies reveal aspartic acid and glutamic acid load on the same receptors in the brain, causing identical brain lesions and neuroendocrine disorders and act in an additive fashion. People who are sensitive to processed free glutamic acid (MSG) experience similar reactions to aspartame, and people who are sensitive to aspartame experience similar reactions to MSG. People who currently react to MSG and/or aspartame should expect to react similarly to neotame. Found in soft drinks, pharmaceuticals, processed foods of all kinds.

Nitrate/Nitrite

While nitrate itself is harmless, it is readily converted to nitrite. When nitrite combines with compounds called secondary amines, it forms nitrosamines: extremely powerful, cancer-causing chemicals. The chemical reaction occurs most readily at the high temperatures of frying. Nitrite has long been suspected as being a cause of stomach cancer.

Nitrosamines

Extremely powerful, cancer-causing chemicals formed at high temperatures when the preservative nitrite combines with compounds called secondary amines.

Olestra

While fat-free, this additive has a fatal side effect: it attaches to valuable nutrients and flushes them out of the body. Some of these nutrients, called carotenoids, appear to protect us from such diseases as lung cancer, prostate cancer, heart disease, and macular degeneration. Olestra replaces fats in "fat-free" foods.

Padimate O (PABA)

Nitrosamines, potent carcinogens may form in products that contain padimate O. There is no way of knowing if they have formed. Found in cosmetics and sunscreens.

Paraffin

Possible carcinogen. Found in cosmetics and food.

PBDE
Toxic flame retardant used in baby bedding to slow advance of fire. Residue found in breast milk.

Perchlorate
Perchlorate is a by-product of rocket fuel, discovered in over 90 percent of the U.S. lettuce and milk supply. It interferes with thyroid function and can cause thyroid cancer and or hypothyroidism.

PEG Stearates
Potentially contaminated with or breaking down into chemicals causing cancer or other significant health problems. Found in cosmetics, creams, and foods.

PEG (Polyethylene, polyethylene glycol, polyoxyethylene, oxynol: any ethoxylated compound, including SLES)

May contain ¼ dioxane, which is a possible carcinogen; estrogen mimic and endocrine disruptor. Can only be removed from a product through vacuum stripping during processing. Avoid all ethyoxylated products as a precaution. Found in foods and body products.

PEG-12 Distearate
May contain harmful impurities or form toxic breakdown products linked to cancer or other significant health problems. Found in creams, lotions, cosmetics, and foods.

PEG-80 Sorbitan Laurate
May contain harmful impurities or form toxic breakdown products linked to cancer or other significant health problems, gastrointestinal or liver toxicity hazards. Found in cosmetics, creams, lotions, and foods.

PEG-14M
May contain harmful impurities or form toxic breakdown products linked to cancer or other significant health problems. Found in foods, lotions, creams, and cosmetics.

Petroleum (Petrolatum)

Suffocates skin and traps toxins in body, clogs pores. Found in lotions, skin creams, and body jelly.

PFOA or C8

Used when processing polytetrafluroroethylene (PTFE) or Teflon. This toxic chemical remains in animals and humans for indefinite periods.

PFOS

Perfluorooctanotane sulfonate. A fluorocarbon used in producing repellants and surfactant products, like stain-resistant fabric.

Phenoxyethanol

Possible connection to reproductive or developmental harm to fetus, potential for reduced fertility, classified as toxic and an irritant, potential risks to wildlife and environment through excretion of body product toxins and disposal of cosmetics.

Phthalates

Accumulates in the body; proven damage to liver, lungs, kidneys, and reproductive systems. Appears in vinyl flooring, plastic wallpaper, perfume, hair spray, deodorant, nail polish, hair gel, mousse, and body and hand lotion. Look for it in children's toys as DEHP, BBP, and DBP.

Polyethylene Glycol /PEG

Moderately toxic, eye irritant, and possible carcinogen. Many glycols produce severe acidosis and cause central nervous system damage and congestion. Can cause convulsions, mutations, and surface EEG changes. Found in cosmetics, body products, foods, lotions.

Polypropylene

Possible carcinogen. Found in lipstick, mascara, baby soap, eye shadow.

Polyscorbate-60
Used in cosmetics. Inhalation could cause chemical pneumonitis.

Polyquaternium-7
May contain harmful impurities or form toxic breakdown products linked to cancer or other significant health problems. Found in body products.

Potassium Bromate
An additive that increases the volume and crumb of bread is banned worldwide except in the United States and Japan. Considered carcinogenic.

p-Phenylenediamine (PPD)
Very toxic substance used in hair dyeing, shampoos, and hair spray. Highly carcinogenic; causes developmental and reproductive toxicity. It is allergenic and can cause skin irritation issues.

Propylene Glycol
Causes kidney damage and liver abnormalities, inhibits skin cell growth, damages cell membranes causing rashes, surface damage, and dry skin.

Absorbed into bloodstream and travels to all organs. Many glycols produce severe acidosis, central nervous system damage, and congestion. Can cause convulsions, mutations, and surface EEG changes. It is derived from petroleum products. The Material Safety Data Sheets on propylene glycol warns against contact with eyes, skin, and clothing. It also says inhalation can cause irritation of nasal passages; ingestion can cause nausea, vomiting, and diarrhea.

Research also shows that it alters cell membranes and causes cardiac arrest. Found in shaving gel, lotions, shampoo, conditioners, foods, deodorant.

Propylparaben

Potential breast cancer risk and endocrine disruptor, raising concern for impaired fertility or development and increased risk for certain cancers; causes itching, burning, and blistering of skin; gastrointestinal or liver toxicity hazard. A close cousin of benzoic acid: poisonous and moderately toxic. Found in body products.

PVC/ Polyvinyl Chloride

When produced or burned, this common plastic releases dioxins that may cause cancer and affect immune and reproductive systems.

Quaternium-7, 15, 31, 60, etc.

Toxic; causes skin rashes and allergic reactions. Formaldehyde releasers. Substantive evidence of casual relation to leukemia, multiple myeloma, non-Hodgkin's lymphoma, and other cancers. Found in body products.

Sodium Chloride

Table salt (processed at high heat). Causes eye irritation, some hair loss, and dry and itchy skin. Found in shampoo as a thickener.

Sodium Hydroxymethylglycinate

Potentially contaminated with or broke down into chemicals linked to cancer or other significant health problems. Found in facial moisturizer, facial cleanser, facial treatments, skin fading and lightening products, anti-aging products, eye makeup remover, concealer, makeup remover, around-eye cream, acne treatment, shampoo, conditioner, styling lotion and gel, styling mousse and foam, hair spray, hair relaxer, tanning oil and sunscreen, after-tanning products, body cleanser and wash, body exfoliants, body firming lotion, baby soap, baby lotion, baby wipes, baby bubble bath, pain and wound products, hand sanitizer.

Sodium Nitrite

Makes meat look red rather than gray and gives meat an overly long shelf life of months. Clinically proven to cause leukemia, brain tumors, and other forms of cancer.

Soy

Contains several naturally occurring compounds that are toxic to humans and animals. Soy foods block calcium and can cause vitamin D deficiencies. One health agency estimates that 100 grams of soy protein provides the estrogenic equivalent of the pill. Processed and all modern soy foods contain MSG, which cause neurological problems. Soy products inhibit thyroid function, which may lead to fatigue and mental issues. Infants on soy formula are vulnerable to developing autoimmune thyroid disease when exposed to high amounts of isoflavones over time. These isoflavones have been found to have serious health effects, including infertility, thyroid disease, or liver disease, on a number of mammals. Long-term feeding with soy formulas inhibits thyroid peroxidase to such an extent that long-term elevated thyroid stimulating hormone levels can also raise the risk of thyroid cancer. It is said that two glasses of soy milk a day over the course of a month contains enough of the chemical to change the timing of a woman's menstrual cycle. Only eat soy if it has been fermented, such as soy, misu and tamari, and if it is labeled as organic or non-GMO.

SLS (Sodium Lauryl Sulphate)

Builds up in heart, lungs, brain, and liver from skin contact and may cause damage to these organs. Corrodes hair follicles and may cause hair to fall out. Damages immune system. Contains endocrine disruptors and estrogen mimics. Impairs proper structural formation of young eyes. May contain carcinogenic nitrosamines. This is a detergent derived from coconut oil and may be labeled natural or even organic. Found in toothpaste, soap, shampoo, body wash, bubble bath, facial cleansers.

SLES (Sodium Laureth Sulfate)

Ether mixtures may contain carcinogenic nitrosamines. Avoid ethoxylated compounds as a precaution. May form 1.4 dioxane, a potential carcinogen, endocrine disruptor, and estrogen mimic. Allows other chemicals to penetrate skin more deeply and enter bloodstream. May cause hair loss when applied to scalp. Found in shampoo, toothpaste, bubble bath, body wash, soap.

Stearalkonium Chloride

Toxic and causes allergic reactions. Used in hair conditioners.

Sulfites

Can cause reactions in asthmatics and can lead to death. Sulphites are now banned on all foods except raw potatoes, wines, and dried fruit.

Talc

Carcinogenic when inhaled, may result in fallopian tube fibrosis. Found in blush, condoms, baby powder, feminine powders, foot and body powders.

Thimerol

At one time found in most vaccines for children. Still believed to be in many vaccines. This form of organic mercury functions as a preservative. It is highly toxic as it metabolizes into methylmercury.

TEA: Tea, Triethanolamine

Tea causes allergic reactions including eye problems, dryness of hair and skin, and could be toxic if absorbed into the body over a long period of time. These chemicals are already restricted in Europe due to known carcinogenic effects (although still in use in the United States).

Repeated skin applications of DEA-based detergents resulted in a major increase in the incidence of liver and kidney cancer. Found in shampoos, skin cream, bubble bath, shaving gel, conditioner, lotions.

Toluene

Poison to humans. Causes hallucinations, bone marrow changes. May also cause liver and kidney damage and birth defects. A known endocrine disruptor and potential carcinogen linked to brain cancer. Irritates respiratory tract. Found in nail polish and cleaning products.

Triclosan

Found in a lot of antimicrobial soaps and toothpaste products, it can react with chlorine in the tap water to create chloroform. This is a toxic chemical that can give you cancer. If you breathe enough chloroform, you will die. When you wash your hands with antibacterial soap that contains triclosan, you are getting the fumes emitted from this chemical reaction.

Vinyl Chloride

Used to create PVC (polyvinyl chloride), a known carcinogen. Often found in toys. Children chewing on toys can release toxins into their bodies.

Zinc Stearate

Carcinogen. Found in blush and powder foundation.

Shamefully, our planet is getting sicker and sicker. Random chemical analysis and laboratory tests of the fluids and gases of the earth show there are toxic chemicals everywhere. These chemicals are affecting every living organism. Nutritional deficiencies along with toxic chemicals are stressing our health. We are hurting ourselves with the same chemicals that we invented to make life easier.

CHAPTER 4

THE IMPLICATIONS OF
RADIATION FALLOUT

Nuclear weapon testing was conducted in the open atmosphere at numerous sites between 1945 and 1980. The United States, the USSR, the UK, France and China carried out more than five hundred atmospheric tests, which resulted in the radioactive exposures to worldwide populations. The nuclear tests were conducted at primarily sixteen sites located in nine different countries on five continents. There were large differences in the number and kinds of tests conducted at each location and in the total explosive yields. Those factors, as well as the differences in the population density, lifestyle, environment and climate at each site, led to large differences in the doses received by local populations. Local, intermediate and global fallout deposition densities downwind from the test sites depended on the heights of the bursts, the yields and the half-lives of the radioactive isotopes. Unfortunately, radioactive fallout drifted across most of the globe and unsuspecting citizens were never adequately warned or told what precautions to take.

Although evaluating the radiation exposures is difficult, the fission and fusion products released have been determined. These tests resulted in the release of substantial quantities of radioactive debris to the environment. The Natural Resources Defense Council estimated that the U.S. bomb tests alone from 1945 to 1962 released the 137,000 kilotons of explosive power. The Soviet Union alone accounted for over 402,000 kilotons.

Dividing these figures by the estimated power of the Hiroshima bomb yields the fact that the superpowers subjected the populations of the world to the fallout of over forty thousand Hiroshima bombs. Microscopic, radioactive isotopes circulated in the air and eventually settled into the ground and the water. Once radioactive fission products come down in the rain and enter the food chain, immune systems become susceptible to the effects of fallout. There is little doubt that high-dose radiation exposure can cause cancer. These highly toxic charged free radicals destroy cell membranes, which causes cancer. This has become clear from studies of groups such as the survivors of the atomic blasts in Japan where the risks of certain cancers were higher than normal.

Public concerns have been raised regarding the lack of information on the potential health risks, lack of warning and lack of oversight. Most funding regarding exposure to fallout has been for research-related activities rather than addressing the health care of exposed individuals. Concerns and complaints are rooted in the government secrecy surrounding the development and testing of nuclear weapons, the withheld government information about radiation health risks and the imposition of past exposures without informed consent. Unfortunately, the impact of weapons fallout will continue to be felt for years to come. If truth be told, the burden and costs of unbridled atomic energy development is overwhelming and is still being calculated. There exists a large body of detailed information concerning the injurious (including lethal) effects of ionizing radiation on numerous animal species studied in the laboratory, as well as upon man. In 1990, the National Research Council published the "Health Effects of Exposure to Low Levels of Ionizing Radiation." It reviews the health risks of radiation-induced cancers, analyzes data in terms of risk estimates for specific organs in relation to dose and time after exposure, and compares radiation effects between Japanese and Western populations. There have been other studies of radiation effects by the U.S. Department of Energy, the National Cancer Institute and the National Academy of Science.

In the last fifty years, there have been numerous governments and independent reports researching the effects of radiation on humans and the environment. The Radiation Effects Research Foundation (REFR) is a cooperative Japan-U.S. Research Organization. It has studied the early, late and genetic effects on atomic bomb survivors. The National Cancer Institute Study Estimating Thyroid Doses of I-131 Received by Americans from Nevada Atmospheric Nuclear Bomb Test was made available to the public in 1997. The Off-Site Radiation Exposure and Review Project (ORERP) was performed from 1979 to 1987 to calculate the external and internal doses from the nuclear weapons tests. Although the study reconstructed the doses from radionuclides, it was unable to clearly define any recommendations or remedies for the effected people. In 1991, the International Physicians for the Prevention of Nuclear War published their study, "Radioactive Heaven and Earth." In 2003, the National Research Council made a review of the CDC-NCI report on the "Exposure of the American Population to Radioactive Fallout from Nuclear Weapons Tests." In 2005, Department of Health and Human Services transmitted to Congress a very long technical report on "A Feasibility Study on the Health Consequences to the American Population from Nuclear Weapons Tests Conducted by the United States and Other Nations." The 2006, January/February issue of *American Scientist* detailed "Fallout from Nuclear Weapons Tests and Cancer Risks," explaining how exposures fifty years ago still have health implications today that will continue into the future. In 2006, the United Nations Scientific Committee on the Effects of Atomic Radiation issued its report on the, "Effects of Ionizing Radiation," summarizing and evaluating sources of human radiation exposures.

Just as the leukemia rates in Japan rose sharply by 50 percent between 1946 and the early 1950s, the same was true in America just ten years later as a result of nuclear bomb testing. There were rises in infant mortality and children born with congenital defects that closely followed the radiation fallout. For young people of both sexes, white and nonwhite alike, there were sudden jumps in the cancer rates between 1948 and 1951. Statistics indicate that radiation was the dominant factor in changes of mortality trends. The fallout from tens of millions of pounds of radioactive isotopes circling the world in matter of a few weeks was especially injurious to the developing young and the very old. Those with weak immune systems were especially vulnerable to the radioactivity. Some other effects of "permissible" low-level radiation include low birth weight babies, mental retardation, and respiratory diseases. In addition, radioactive fallout has been linked with the declining learning and reading ability scores of young students born in the 1950s.

The leading long-term hazard associated with ionizing radiation is increased cancer rates. When there were nuclear explosions, the spontaneous emission of beta and gamma rays from the disintegration of the nuclei of atoms produced much harm—the most serious being the altering of the genetic makeup of cells. Many of these radioactive elements got into the ground and the water and were eventually ingested through foodstuffs. These highly charged free radicals destroy cell membranes, which lead to malignant cells. A range of diseases can be traced to the genetic altering of chromosomes. Most of these radioactive ions may be expected to produce abnormal molecules that can cause the cell to proliferate into a cancerous growth. What's more, low-level radiation has done more damage to wildlife and plants than initially believed.

The effects of fallout radiation in causing leukemia and other cancers in persons is a foregone conclusion with delayed effects appearing months or years later. Some of the possible delayed consequences of radiation injury are life shortening, carcinogenesis, decreased fertility and genetic mutations. Even very low doses of radiation pose a risk of cancer over a person's lifetime. However, cancer effects from acute exposure usually appear quickly. If the radiation dose is high, there is extensive cell damage, and the health effects are seen immediately. Acute health effects include burns and radiation sickness. The symptoms of radiation sickness include nausea, weakness, hair loss, skin burns and diminished organ function. Vomiting and diarrhea are caused by doses above 50 rads. Penetrating radiation doses above 100 rads inflicts severe skin burns. Doses of 1,000 rads or more would cause paralysis of the central nervous system and immediate brain death. Then there are the long-term health effects of teratogenic and genetic mutations. Genetic effects are those that can be passed from parent to child. Teratogenic mutations result from the exposure of fetuses (unborn children) to radiation. These can include smaller head or brain size, poorly formed eyes, abnormally slow growth and mental retardation.

The rays of gamma radiation are like little bullets that shoot through the body. They tear electrons away from the molecules and, through subsequent reactions of the molecular ions that are formed the molecules may be broken into two. Some atoms may be torn away and new molecules may be formed. The exposure of the human body to 1 roentgen of radiation causes about a thousand ions to be formed in each cell of the human body. The most important molecules affected are the DNA that governs the behavior of the cell. DNA controls the manufacture of other molecules and the process by which the cell divides to form new cells. This is the reason that there is no safe amount of radiation or of radioactive material. Even small amounts do harm. When the exposure is large, there is no doubt that ionizing radiation produces cancer.

High-level radiation includes alpha particles, beta particles, neutrons, x-rays, and gamma rays. Alpha and beta rays are fast-moving particles emitted by the decomposing radioactive nuclei. Gamma rays are rays of penetrating radiation identical in nature to x-radiation. The gamma rays from radioactive nuclei are highly penetrating and can pass completely through the human body, irradiating all parts of it. Internal irradiation exposures can arise from inhaling fallout and absorbing it through intact or injured skin, but the main exposure route is from consumption of contaminated food. Vegetation can be contaminated when fallout is directly deposited on external surfaces of plants and when it is absorbed through the roots of plants. The lethal impact of ingesting fission products may continue to persist throughout a person's lifetime.

The mostly commonly encountered radionuclides from fallout include the following:

Name	Atomic Number	Alpha	Beta	Gamma
americium-241	95	x		x
cesium-137	55		x	x
cobalt-60	27		x	x
iodine-129 and -131	53		x	x
plutonium	94	x	x	x
radium	88	x		x
radon	86	x		
strontium-90	38		x	
technetium-99	43		x	x
tritium	1		x	
thorium	90	x		x
uranium	92	x		x

Everyone in the world is now receiving some additional exposure from fallout. Radionuclides from nuclear fallout include iodine, cesium, strontium, barium, ruthenium, tellurium, uranium and plutonium. Radioactive debris injected into the stratosphere takes time to deposit, during which time the shorter-lived radionuclides largely disappear through radioactive decay. Of greater concern are two longer-lived radionuclides, strontium-90 and cesium-137, which have thirty-year half-lives and therefore cause the most harm. The radioactive materials in the stratosphere fall to the ground very slowly. Almost 50 percent may remain in the stratosphere after fifteen years. The winds in the stratosphere have time to distribute these radioactive materials nearly uniformly over the surface of the earth. During these years, most of the radioactive nuclei with small half-lives decompose. Those with large half-lives in large part remain undecomposed and retain their activity when they reach the surface of the earth even after twenty years or more. Strontium and cesium have introduced a biological hazard to the environment, and as a result, almost every living person carries both these radionuclides. Our foodstuffs, grown on soil contaminated with both of these long-persisting radionuclides, are essentially contaminated by them.

Another related carcinogen, neutron radiation, can be released by nuclear fusion or fission of atomic nuclei in nuclear reactors or atomic explosions. Neutrons are also known to cause genetic damage in humans. Studies of humans exposed to neutron radiation showed that induced chromosomal aberrations persisted for decades, and some cell-culture studies showed genomic instability in the progeny of irradiated human cells. There is also sufficient evidence of carcinogenicity from studies in experimental animals. Neutrons cause ionization in biological tissue through elastic collisions with the nuclei of atoms composing tissue molecules.

In all probability, all forms of human cancer are induced by ionizing radiation. The question is how much damage will be produced to the immune systems per extra rad of radiation delivered. After tissue is exposed to radiation, the initial radiation scatters, and atoms in the body are ionized by removal of weakly bound electrons. Ionizing radiation and certain chemicals can produce both single-strand breaks and double-stand breaks in the DNA backbone.

The U.S. Department of Health and Human Services National Toxicology's Program's annual report points out the clear dangers of ionizing radiation. The report states that x-radiation and gamma radiation cause a broad spectrum of genetic damage, including gene mutation, micronucleus formation, sister chromatid exchange, chromosomal aberrations, DNA strand breaks and chromosomal instability. Although the radiation that will affect the probability of cancer is dependent on the dose and the dose rate, there is no safe level of exposure. Genetic damage by x-radiation and gamma radiation has been observed in humans exposed accidentally, occupationally or environmentally. The DNA molecule may be damaged directly or indirectly by interaction with ionizing radiation. If the cell is exposed to ionizing radiation, double-stranded breaks occur along the entire length of the DNA. Mutations occur if the repair mechanisms re-attach the wrong piece of DNA back together so that a part of the DNA strand goes missing. This may lead to the deletion of important genes or a change in the location of a gene within the DNA. These types of mutations are linked to the development of a number of cancers, including leukemia, bone, lung and breast cancer. The observed genetic damage is primarily the result of errors in DNA repair but may also arise from errors in replication of damaged DNA.

The effect of high-energy radiation in causing mutations and chromosomal damage has significantly damaged the human gene pool. Geneticists also believe that the number of mutations in human beings caused by radiation is proportional to the amount to radiation that reaches the gonads. Almost all major diseases afflicting man are in part caused by damage to the genetic material of the ova or sperm. Atomic radiation poses genetic hazards where radiation delivered to the ovary of women and testis of men damages the germ plasm of future generations. There is considerable evidence that radiation exposure affects the embryonic neuronal system. The causes of early death as a result of radiation exposure are complex, depending on the radiation dose and the length of exposure. Nuclear radiation arises from hundreds of different kinds of unstable atoms. Ionizing radiation, which can damage living tissue, is emitted as the unstable atoms (radionuclides) change spontaneously to become different types of atoms.

Many species of animals have been thoroughly tested and all have been found to have an increase in mutation rate upon exposure to ionizing radiation. The primary concern is that tests of nuclear weapons have produced mutations in the genes of human beings, such that there will be an increase in the number of defective children born in later generations. Even a 1 percent increase in the number of bad genes means a tragedy for many human beings. The number of children born with gross physical and mental defects will appear in many future generations as a result of the atomic bomb tests. Mutant genes that cause diabetes, hemophilia, muscular dystrophy, microcephaly, and many other diseases are increased by fallout radioactivity. This does not include embryonic and neonatal deaths and stillbirths attributed to the bomb tests. There is no doubt that small amounts of radiation received from fallout radioactivity can cause gene mutation that increases the number of defective children born in future generations. The fact remains that the testing of nuclear weapons was inadvertently carried out at the expense of the lives of children as yet unborn therefore it may even do irreversible harm to posterity.

The scope of the problem is immense, yet the majority of people are not aware of the grave dangers of nuclear pollution. Incredibly, this understanding has either been ignored or overlooked even though it could be considered the world's number one environmental hazard. Cancer rates have increased because appreciable quantities of radioactivity continue to find its way into the environment. A somewhat short-sighted nuclear weapons industry has been endangering the lives of its citizens in the name of national security. For years, private contractors ran the major U.S. weapons plants and nuclear power plants that released huge quantities of radioactive particles into the air and dumped tons of potentially cancer-inducing refuse into flowing creeks and leaking pits, contaminating underground water supplies. Since the 1950s, the defense industry has deposited over 120,000 drums of low-level radiation waste in different places on a "temporary" basis.

There have been many studies to assess radiation damage, but no one really knows how many people may have been needlessly afflicted with such ailments as cancer, birth deformities, and thyroid deficiencies. Nuclear reactor accidents, like Three Mile Island in 1979, Chernobyl in 1986, and Fukushima in 2011, only increase cancer risks. On April 26, 1986, the nuclear reactor accident at Chernobyl released hundreds of millions of curies of radiation into the biosphere. The resulting fallout was felt thousands of miles away, and significant increases in death were recorded in the Ukraine and in Europe. The Fukushima Daiichi nuclear power plant has been leaking considerable radiation since March 11, 2011. The earthquake and tsunami disabled power and cooling systems which led to three meltdowns and forced 160,000 people to flee their homes. The Fukushima prefecture has a high level of radioactive contamination that will make that area unusable for generations. There have been thirty-three serious accidents since 1952 where large quantities of radioactivity were released into the atmosphere. A nuclear reactor can release radioactive isotopes with a longer half-life than that of a nuclear bomb. Presently, there are over 432 nuclear power plants in the world with another 65 under construction. There has been much secrecy and classified information withheld, yet the consequences of the radioactive fallout from the nuclear industry is all around us.

If truth be told, there are a wide range of government agencies and regulatory departments that try to protect its citizens from harmful radiation including:

1. the Department of Energy
2. the Department of Health and Human Services
3. the Department of Transportation
4. the Environmental Protection Agency
5. the Food and Drug Administration
6. the Nuclear Regulatory Commission
7. the Occupational Safety and Health Administration
8. the American Conference of Government Industrial Hygienists
9. the Food and Drug Administration
10. the National Institute for Occupational Safety and Health
11. the National Toxicology Program
12. the Agency for Toxic Substances and Disease Registry
13. the National Academies of Science's Biological Effects of Ionizing Radiation Report Series
14. the International Agency for Research on Cancer
15. National Council on Radiation Protection and Measurements
16. United Nations Scientific Committee on the Effects of Atomic Radiation
17. the International Commission on Radiological Protection

There are also non-government agencies dealing with the effects of ionizing radiation which include the American Cancer Society, the Centers for Disease Control, the World Health Organization, the National Council on Radiation Protection and Measurements and the Conference of Radiation Control Program. For decades, the National Cancer Institute has been studying groups of people who were exposed to ionizing radiation from nuclear accidents and above ground atomic weapons explosions to learn about the cancer risks from these exposures. This enormous amount of scientific research will help minimize the effects of future nuclear accidents, but they have yet to find the remedy for radiation effects. In fact, man-made sources of radiation (e.g., television, computer screens, cell phones, electromagnetic fields, microwaves, medical imaging, and airline travel) add to the amount of radiation the average person can contend with. Moreover, the use of ionizing radiation(chemo) as a cancer treatment has been a contradiction in terms. If the doctors really knew that the cancer was caused by radiation, they wouldn't treat it so. The harmful side effects from chemotherapy radiation alone is distressing.

The radiation from power lines and electrical objects that surround us daily is considered by some in the scientific community to cause comparable symptoms as chemical toxins. Research links this modern bombardment from even low-level frequencies to brain cancer and miscarriages. The risk estimates, the medical data, the analytical studies all point to an increased radiation problem of mammoth proportions. This does not include the possibility of human devastation from bio-terrorist attacks, the mismanagement of nuclear waste, and the most unthinkable—the actual use of nuclear weapons.

CHAPTER 5

THE MEDICAL SYSTEM IS FAILING

M edical science and technology are advancing rapidly. The genetic code has been broken, nanotechnology is becoming pervasive and robots are performing surgery. However, a large majority of people have either high cholesterol or high blood pressure, or both. Unfortunately, the more technologically advanced we develop, the sicker we become. There are more dedicated workers in the health care sector than in any other part of the economy. Yet, infectious diseases are spreading around the world faster than ever, and new diseases are emerging at the unprecedented rate of one per year. Chronic diseases are on the rise, more and more patients are on antidepressants, and this is occurring at higher rates in industrialized countries than in developing nations. In fact, diseases seem to be affecting younger and younger patients all the time. Thousands of people die every year from the side effects of improperly prescribed medications and failed medical treatments. Drugs today may be causing more harm than the problems they are supposed to solve. The once-formidable traditional medical foundation is starting to collapse from the weight of its own ignorance of alternatives, greed for money, and medical mistakes. The present system of high-powered prescription medication and advanced surgery does not have impressive results. Even though the amount of money that is spent in the prevention and treatment of disease is mind-boggling, medical expenses are rising faster than the costs of any other service. A Harvard University study found that up to 50 percent of personal bankruptcies in the United States are due to medical costs. The cost of health care is unmanageable because the focus is more on disease management than on prevention and health promotion. One of the biggest paradoxes in the world is the fact that the present health care system, is unhealthy. It is unfair, expensive, and badly in need of reform.

Medical malpractice has become the third leading cause of death in the United States, after deaths from heart disease and cancer. Emergency room errors have led to serious complications from medication overdoses, wrong diagnostic testing and infections due to unsanitary conditions. A statistical study of hospital deaths in the United States conducted at the University of Toronto revealed that pharmaceutical drugs kill more people every year than traffic accidents. What's more, studies have shown that medical errors rates are underreported. Roughly one of three people encounters an adverse event when they are admitted to a hospital. Negligently performed surgeries, misdiagnosis and mistaken medications continue on a daily basis. The individuals who are most at risk are the ones who can least afford to become ill, sick individuals already in the hospital, and those with a compromised immune system. There is an ever-increasing danger of infections that are resistant to most if not all antibiotics. Physicians do not always have an effective treatment plan in place. Even with today's modern medicine, thousands of people die because of blood poisoning in hospitals called sepsis. Another serious problem is Methicillin-resistant *Staphylococcus aureus* (MRSA). This is a type of staph bacteria that does not respond to some antibiotics that are commonly used to treat staph infections. Part of the problem is the relative unknown nature of these illnesses as more and more deadly pathogens are becoming drug resistant.

Many people think of hospitals as places where they and their loved ones go to get well. However, statistics support a growing concern that patients are contracting infections and disease while being treated in hospitals, leading to further injury, illness or even death. The Center for Disease Control estimates that hospital-acquired infections account for 1.7 million infections and 99,000 deaths annually. All hospitalized patients are at risk. Medical errors and the problems they can cause—including bed sores, post-op infections, and implant or device complications—cost the U.S. economy $19.5 billion in 2008. Antibiotics, which are used to treat virtually every malady, are often unnecessary, inappropriate, or of no value. Deaths from overdose of prescription painkillers have skyrocketed in the past decade. Every year, nearly fifteen thousand people die from overdose involving these drugs—more than those who die from heroin and cocaine combined. Nearly half a million emergency department visits in 2009 were due to people misusing or abusing prescription painkillers. Annual drug overdose deaths are approaching the same number of people killed in automobile accidents, the leading cause of injurious death.

Class action lawsuits against drug companies and hospital mistakes cost millions every year. Prescription drugs cause serious harmful side effects even without the medical errors. One in seven patients suffers harm, mostly from oversedation. Medication errors include errors involving the wrong drug, wrong dose, wrong patient, wrong time, wrong rate, wrong preparation, or wrong route of administration. Other harmful side effects include depression, nausea, insomnia, headaches, rapid heartbeat and even suicide. This leads to psychological and social problems as well. Abusing prescription drugs leads to addiction and crime, including pharmacy robberies.

Surgical errors, misdiagnosis cases, and other instances of medical malpractice are more widespread than previously believed. Some patients adversely affected by the actions or neglect of a doctor or hospital pursue their cases and find justice, but many never even know or understand that they are victims of medical malpractice. Regarding medical malpractice:

- An estimated 225,000 people die each year from some form of medical malpractice, from incorrect dosages to surgical errors to wrong diagnosis. This is the third most common reason for death in the United States.
- Only 2 percent of those who suffer from medical malpractice ever file claims for compensation. Even fewer ever receive compensation for their injury, failing health, pain or suffering.
- The *Journal of the American Medical Association* reports that 106,000 patients die each year because of the negative effects of their medication.
- The Institute of Medicine estimates that medication errors are the most common of medical errors, with 1.5 million people suffering injury from these mistakes each year.

Common complaints against doctors include failure or error to diagnose correctly, acquired infections and incorrectly performed procedures. These errors are becoming increasingly common as medical care becomes more complex, with miscommunication and systemic problems at the root of many failures.

The way our medical system works today, drug companies are the primary entities that fund research test and prepare medical treatments for government approval. However, simple, inexpensive and safer medicines are not promoted because they are not good for drug company's profits. It is the drug industry's best interest to ignore and invalidate medicines and traditional therapies that can't be patented and don't produce a large profit. There are numerous studies proving the effectiveness, safety and diverse medical applications of alternative therapies, yet most conventional doctors will tell you that they are unscientific and ineffective. Doctors tell you this because their medical training is completely centered around drug and surgery treatments promoted by the pharmaceutical industry. Synthetic drugs, unlike herbs or other simple medicines, can be patented and sold for enormous profits. If an alternative therapy is not picked up by a drug company and presented for government approval, the general public will probably never learn or receive the benefits, no matter how good they are.

The "war on cancer" is actually being fought against alternative cancer treatments. Cancer patients deserve to make choices based upon all the information available. Already, there are proven cancer prevention strategies and real cures. They do not need a prescription, nor do they require surgery or harsh procedures like radiation and chemotherapy. Doctors are afraid their insurance carrier may drop them if they use alternative treatments. Their state medical boards may fine them and revoke their license. Due to the fact that others doctors will publicly ridicule them if they use alternative treatments, many doctors succumb to peer pressure. Doctors are against these treatments because from the first day of medical school, they are convinced that cancer can only be treated with drugs, chemo, surgery and radiation-even though less than 1/3 of the over-the-counter drug ingredients have been shown to be safe and effective for their intended uses.

With the increasing population, there are too many people in too many places for the existing medical establishment to handle. Therefore alternative or integrative methods are the best bet to cure illnesses. Some of these alternatives are based on historical or cultural traditions rather than current scientific evidence. Some are integrating eastern and western medicinal treatments including metaphysical healing in search of cures. Whatever the case may be, the time has finally come for safe, innovative remedies to rejuvenate medical standards.

CHAPTER 6

THE SOLUTION

Urine therapy is a natural, alternative medicine that is incredibly—free. Despite being relatively unknown, this panacea has been empirically proven to be tremendously effective in dealing with all kinds of diseases. It is not glorified by the media nor endorsed by the medical community. It is usually greeted with an initial skepticism, distaste and even shock. Most people do not know (or want to know) anything about the history, testimonies or ingredients of this unrecognized natural medicine. It has gone in and out of vogue since ancient times and yet still remains hidden behind a cloak of secrecy. To understand about this "homemade" medicine it is crucial to be familiar with how the kidneys work. Urine is made in and by our kidneys in a system so complex that researchers still can't completely figure it out. A diagram of the urinary system shows clearly that it is not connected to the intestines or the stomach but comes straight from the blood, through the kidneys and then out the urethra.

The function of the kidneys is not excretion, but regulation. Urine is a by-product of blood filtration, not waste filtration. The kidneys keep the composition of the blood in optimal balance. They filter the elements that need to go back into the bloodstream. Then if the body does not need an element of a particular concentration, it filters them out through the bladder.

THE URINARY SYSTEM

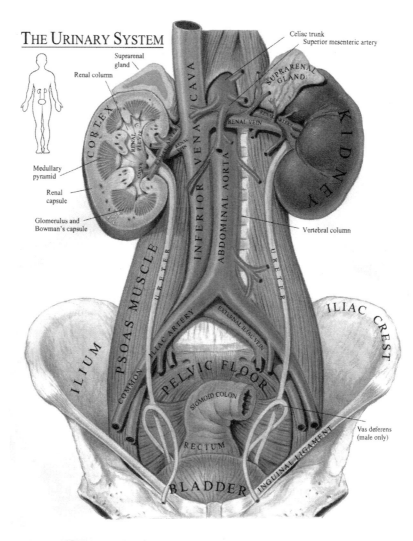

Celiac trunk
Superior mesenteric artery

Suprarenal gland

Renal column

SUPRARENAL GLAND

CORTEX

RENAL VEIN

INFERIOR VENA CAVA

ABDOMINAL AORTA

KIDNEY

Medullary pyramid

RENAL PELVIS

Renal capsule

Glomerulus and Bowman's capsule

Vertebral column

PSOAS MUSCLE

URETER

URETER

COMMON ILIAC ARTERY

EXTERNAL ILIAC VEIN

ILIAC CREST

ILIUM

PELVIC FLOOR

SIGMOID COLON

Vas deferens (male only)

RECTUM

INGUINAL LIGAMENT

BLADDER

The urinary system consists of two kidneys, each with a ureter conveying urine from the kidneys to a collecting sac called the bladder, and a pipe, the urethra, leading to the exterior. The bean-shaped kidneys, 4¼ inches (11 centimeters) long and 1⅛ inches (3 centimeters) thick, lie on either side of the spine, level with the upper lumbar vertebrae. Inside lies a pale outer cortex and a darker medulla composed of tubules leading into a collecting space called the renal pelvis. Kidney tissue is composed of over one million coiled tubules called nephrons. Each begins in the cortex as a cup-shaped Bowman's capsule, containing a tuft of capillaries known as a glomerulus.

Convolutions increase the length of a nephron, and a large loop bends back into the cortex to meet more capillaries from the renal artery, before ending in the medulla. Thus, blood passes through two sets of capillaries in one organ, something that occurs nowhere else in the body. Waste products are filtered out at high pressure—about 162 fluidrams (600 milliliters) of blood per minute pass through the kidney—to maintain the balance of chemicals in the blood. To fine-tune this process, chemicals are selectively reabsorbed or secreted in the end tubules to produce urine, composed of 96 percent water and 4 percent salts and waste products.

When the blood enters the kidneys, it is filtered hundreds of times a day through an immensely complex and intricate system of minute tubules called nephrons. Here, the blood is literally filtered and cleansed at high pressure. Researchers have observed that urine, because it is extracted from our blood, contains small amounts of almost all the life-sustaining elements, enzymes, proteins, hormones, antibodies and immunizing agents that our blood contains. It contains thousands of compounds that are specific to the body and are tailored to keep the body from getting out of balance. In one way or another, when the body is sick, it stimulates the kidneys to make the curative remedy. This antidote could be an antibody, if there is an internal infection, or an antiseptic, if there is an external wound. When this urine is reintroduced to the body, the body's immune system is greatly enhanced. It contains the precise combination of substances that the body needs at the time it is produced. Urine therapy can be seen as a form of self-vaccination where certain body substances are reintroduced into the body in small amounts where the immune system is given a chance to react appropriately.

The idea that urine is a poisonous waste product is not based on fact. It has been scientifically proven that, besides water, urine consists mainly of minerals, hormones and enzymes which are not harmful to the body. The body can reuse many of these substances. Urine is simply a healthy liquid that is filtered out of the bloodstream. What at one moment was part of the blood can be found in urine a split second later. Certain substances are then filtered by the kidneys and secreted as raw materials, which can be directly absorbed by the body upon renewed intake by way of drinking or massaging. The kidneys filter hundreds of liters of blood per day. The greatest part of the filtered urine is directly reabsorbed into the blood. The kidney is not intended to remove poisonous substances from the body—the liver, intestines, skin, and exhalation take care of this.

Urine essentially is blood without the blood cells. Urine and the plasma (the liquid portion of the blood) differ only slightly in composition and concentration. Not only is the urine not waste, it is filled with vital, life-giving elements. It contains, in its fresh condition, only those chemicals and compounds of the blood in circulation in each of us already. There is no greater harmless detoxifying agent in the world than urine. It not only purifies the system but also regenerates and builds up old worn-out and even dead tissues. Urine has the ability to rebuild cells, which is the smallest living unit in the human body. No other element but urine can penetrate to the nucleus of the cell where the genetic material is stored. DNA abnormalities can be reinstated when the ions of the person's urine are exchanged with the damaged ones. Many of the compounds in urine are still being researched to understand their importance and potential.

Urine has ions on the molecular level of:

- ✓ all known vitamins
- ✓ hundreds of proteins
- ✓ hundreds of hormones and steroids
- ✓ hundreds of enzymes
- ✓ hundreds of amino acids
- ✓ dozens of antioxidants
- ✓ traces of most elements of the periodic table
- ✓ significant amounts of seven major minerals and tiny quantities of sixty-five trace minerals
- ✓ numerous antibodies to vaccinate and protect all cells in the body from different species of viruses, bacteria, fungi, and parasites that colonize our body and constantly threaten our health.

Primarily, urine substances consist of the following:

Agglutinins and Precipitins – They have a neutralizing effect on polio and other viruses.

Antineoplaston – It prevents selectively the growth of cancer cells without harming the growth of healthy cells.

Allontoin – A nitrogenous crystal substance which helps heal wounds. It is an oxidation product of uric acid. This substance can be found in many skin cream products.

DHEA – This substance prevents obesity, prolongs the lifespan of animals, and offers a possible treatment for anemia, diabetes, and breast cancer in women. DHEA stimulates the growth of bone marrow and increases the production of substances manufactured by bone marrow such as red blood cells, monocytes, macrophages, and lymphocytes.

Gastric Secretory Depressants – These combat the growth of stomach ulcers.

Glucuronic Acid – It is created in the kidneys, liver, and intestinal canal and has an important secretion function.

H-11 – It inhibits the growth of cancer cells and reduces already-existing tumors without disturbing the recovery process.

HUD (Human's Urine Derivative) – The urine derivative shown to have remarkable anti-cancer properties.

Interleukin-1 – This substance has a positive influence on helper cells and inhibiting substances. It can signal the hypothalamus to produce a fever.

3-methyl-glyoxal – It destroys cancer cells.

Prostaglandin – It is a hormonal substance which dilates the blood vessels and lowers blood pressure, relaxes the bronchial muscles, stimulates labor contractions, and a number of other functions relating to metabolism.

Protein Globulins – This contains antibodies against specific allergens; identical to proteins in immunoglobulins of serum (blood).

Proteses – The immunologically active products of allergic reactions.

Retine – The anti-cancer element extracted from urine.

Uric acid – It helps keep "free radical scavengers" (molecules which can cause cancer) under control, combats old age, and even has a tuberculostatic effect.

Inorganic Substances in Urine:

Bicarbonate, chloride, phosphor, sulphur, bromide, fluoride, iodide, rhodanide, kalium, natrium, calcium, magnesium, iron, copper, zinc, cobalt, selenium, arsenium, lead, mercury.

Nitrogen-Containing Substances in Urine:

Nitrogen, urea, creatine, creatinine, guanidine, choline, carnitine, piperidine, spermi-dine, spermine, dopamine, adrenaline, nor-adrenaline, serotonin, tryptamine, amino-levulinic acid, porphyrin, bilirubin, and others.

Amino Acids in Urine:

Alanine, carnosine, glycine, histidine, leucine, lysine, methionine, phenylalanine, serine, tyrosine, valine, hydroxyproline, galactosylhydroxylysine, xylo-sylserine, and others.

Proteins in Urine:

Albumin, haptoglobin, transferring, IgG, IgA, IgM, and others.

Enzymes in Urine:

Lactatdehydrogenase, gamma-glutamyltransferase, alpha-amylase, uropepsinogen, lysozyme, beta-N-acetylglucosaminidase, urokinanse, protease, and others.

Carbohydrates in Urine:

Arabibose, xylose, ribose, fucose, rhamnose, ketopentose, glucose, galactose, mannose, fructose, lactose, saccharose, fucosylglucose, raffinose and others.

Vitamins in Urine:

Thiamine (B1) riboflavin (B2), vitamin B-6, 4-pyridoxic acid, vitamin b-12, biopterine, ascorbic acid, zinc, magnesium, potassium, folic acid, and others.

Hormones in Urine:

Gonadotropin, coricotropin, prolactin, lactogenic hormones, oxytocin, vasopressin, thyroxine, cathecholamin (adrenaline, noradrenaline, dopamine), insulin, erythropoietin, corticosteroids (aldosterone, corticosterone, cortisone), testosterone, progesterone, oestrogen, and others.

Additionally, urine is estimated to have thousands of biochemical compounds. In view of such an array of ingredients, it is easier to understand urine's antibacterial, antifungal, antiviral, antineoplastic, anticonvulsive, and antispasmodic effects.

Key elements of its biochemical action include the following:

- ✓ Supplements the essential nutrients and makes the deficiency of any nutrient in the body.
- ✓ Contains highly active enzymes that have a salutary effect on all the physiological reactions taking place in the body.
- ✓ Contains valuable salts necessary for the body.
- ✓ Contains hormones that are of great benefit to the body.
- ✓ Possesses bactericidal properties. It therefore destroys the diseases causing bacteria in the body, especially those infesting the digestive tract.
- ✓ Augments and sharpens the body's natural powers of resistance to disease.
- ✓ Increases the efficiency of the kidneys because the urea present in urine is diuretic.
- ✓ Strengthens the body and is an elixir that confers longevity.

Urine is the most complex of all body fluids as it can control and regulate every function in the body. Modern research and clinical studies have proven that thousands of critical body chemicals and nutrients end up in our urine. Subsequently, when urine is used medicinally, the correct concentration antibody is produced to respond to that individual's health threat. What most people don't understand is that the brain directs the kidneys to product the right "medicine" that the body needs when it is sick. Modern research and clinical studies have proven that the thousands of critical body chemicals and nutrients that end up in urine reflect the body functions. When reutilized, they act as natural vaccines, antibacterial, antiviral, anticancer agents, hormone balancers and even allergy relievers. Since it so easily accessible, it gives a whole new meaning to the term "free health care." In fact, there is no need to visit a doctor for a diagnosis or a store to buy any products. To its adherents, it has become the ultimate survival tool.

Not only does urine cleanse the body, but it also revitalizes the spirit. It is a liquid of vital elements to support, strengthen and regenerate life. To many, this is totally incomprehensible because it is so unorthodox. But to others, who have tried everything and have nothing to lose, it has been the best-kept medical secret. Most people are astonished when they learn about it and are even more incredulous they hadn't previously heard about it. Many are afraid to try urine therapy because it is not recommended by their physicians. Many medical practitioners say it has not been proven effective. But the truth is that urine therapy is far safer and effective than prescription drugs, and it has no side effects.

Most medical professionals agree that degenerative diseases like cancer, heart disease and arthritis set in due to the accumulation of toxins in the body. Various methods are suggested for removing those toxins, but there is no greater harmless detoxifying agent in the world than urine. It not only purifies the system but it also regenerates and builds up old, worn-out and even dead tissues. The minerals and enzymes that are passed out in the urine can be easily assimilated to help in the process of tissue building and to fight disease. Human urine has strengthening and curative characteristics for many deficiencies. Man's intelligence and spirit cannot comprehend that the body is an extremely advanced system. The kidneys are like an information card which registers the condition of the blood. That is why any doctor that wants to find out what's wrong with a patient does a urinalysis. What they don't know is that when this information gets back to the body, the body can react according to the feedback. It will do this in a precise and accurate way without the conscious mind even being aware.

The urine contains personal characteristic substances and provides the particular information the body needs in order to carry out the healing process as effectively as possible. Urine therapy works both on a mechanistic and on an energetic level. The latter implies that urine, as a holographic substance, can affect all levels of being, from the physical through the electromagnetical fields of the emotions and the mind up to the subtler genetic vibrational information of the soul. In this sense, urine therapy can be seen as one of the divine manifestations of cosmic intelligence. Urine can be considered to contain an exact holographic picture of the body fluids and tissues. The biofeedback of this holographic information by re-ingesting the urine may well inform the energy system in a way which helps restore a disturbed balance. Once the body has been made conscious of urine, the whole organism evaluates it and subsequently updates its own regulating mechanisms. This theory of transmutation implies that the body is capable, through energetic exchange within the body itself, to transmute certain substances or molecules into new ones. Urine's ability to go deep to restructure disturbed DNA is unmatched.

The abnormal growth of cancer cells is believed to the result of an "error" in their genetic mechanism that controls development. The substance in urine called antineoplaston apparently detects cells that are getting out of line and feeds them new information that returns them to normal. Urine therapy enables the body to create its own vaccine. The microorganisms that infect our systems form toxins and endotoxins and stimulate our immunologic system to form antitoxins (antidotes), which are discarded through the urine. When we take it, we force the bacteria to take their own toxin, which is why we say "poison kills poison." Urine therapy creates an autovaccine that has the same elements of our own illness. This creates processes that are antiviral, anti-neoplastic, anti-spasmodic, anti-inflammatory, antifungal, anti-allergenic, anti-convulsive, along with a cardiovascular stimulant, a diuretic and a bactericide. You simply cannot ask for more than that.

CHAPTER 7

TESTIMONIES AND CASE HISTORIES

Urine therapy helps in the maintenance and healing of the many intricate systems of the body including the digestive system, the excretory system, the urinary system, the respiratory system, the circulatory system, the nervous system, the reproductive system and the overall immune system. Many ailments including multiple sclerosis, colitis, lupus, rheumatoid arthritis, cancer, hepatitis, hyperactivity, pancreatic insufficiency, psoriasis, eczema, diabetes, herpes, mononucleosis, adrenal failure and allergies have been relieved through use of this therapy. Amazingly, urine therapy is effective both externally and internally. It can heal many conditions including:

Externally:
- ✓ Rashes
- ✓ Cuts
- ✓ Scrapes
- ✓ Wounds
- ✓ Burns
- ✓ Sores
- ✓ Athlete's foot
- ✓ Eczema
- ✓ Gangrene
- ✓ Infections
- ✓ Insect bites
- ✓ Warts

- ✓ Varicose veins
- ✓ Pimples, acne
- ✓ Baldness
- ✓ Snake bites
- ✓ Insect bites
- ✓ Nail problems
- ✓ Dandruff
- ✓ Athlete's foot
- ✓ Sunburn
- ✓ Eye troubles
- ✓ Ear infections
- ✓ Toothaches
- ✓ Warts
- ✓ Hives
- ✓ Ringworm
- ✓ Glaucoma
- ✓ Psoriasis
- ✓ Fungus
- ✓ Dermatitis

Internally:

- ✓ Cancer
- ✓ Heart disease
- ✓ Diabetes
- ✓ High blood pressure
- ✓ Hormonal imbalances
- ✓ Allergies
- ✓ Constipation
- ✓ Diarrhea
- ✓ Colds and flu symptoms
- ✓ Arthritis
- ✓ Asthma
- ✓ Herpes, venereal diseases

- ✓ Jaundice, hepatitis
- ✓ Mononucleosis
- ✓ Prostrate disorders
- ✓ Rheumatism
- ✓ Sexual impotency
- ✓ Meningitis
- ✓ Hepatitis
- ✓ Tuberculosis
- ✓ Parkinson's disease
- ✓ Food poisoning
- ✓ Gout
- ✓ Lupus
- ✓ Ulcers
- ✓ Parasites
- ✓ Mononucleosis
- ✓ Hepatitis
- ✓ Viruses

The most amazing aspect of urine therapy is its effectiveness in such a wide range of different diseases. This may be from its contents of countless hormones, enzymes, vitamins, trace minerals and other valuable biochemicals. One well-known urine ingredient is melatonin, the hormone of the pineal gland. What's more, urine contains antibodies and immune stimulating factors against all viruses, harmful bacteria or fungi that we may harbor in our body. Even minute amounts of antibodies, sometimes so low they cannot be detected with conventional methods, are effective in preventing and treating diseases. There are various accounts describing the curative effects of urine therapy on a wide range of infections, fungal and viral infections, such as hepatitis, poliomyelitis and AIDS.

Urine is especially effective against allergies, autoimmune diseases and other disorders of the immune system. Cancer, too, responds very well to urine therapy. Most of the scientific cancer reports concentrate on urine extracts of anti-cancer agents. These include H-11, HUD, retine, DHEA hormone and anti-neoplaston. The strongest cancer-fighting ingredient may be urea, the most common element in urine.

Although no scientific research through double blind studies have been done on the importance of urine as a cure-all, there are numerous testimonies that cannot be denied. One notable testimony came from the former prime minister of India, Morarji Desai. He lived to be almost a hundred and testified to the healing properties of urine to anyone who would listen. In 1978, he was interviewed by Dan Rather on *60 Minutes*, and he stated that urine therapy was the perfect medical solution for millions of Indians who cannot afford medical treatment. His book, *Miracles of Urine Therapy*, summarizes its cures.

British actress Sarah Miles has drunk her own urine for over thirty years, claiming that it immunizes against allergies. Major League baseball player Moises Alou urinated on his hands to alleviate calluses, which he claims allows him to bat without using batting gloves. Singer/actress Madonna explained to talk show host David Letterman that she urinates on her feet to help cure her athlete's foot. Alternative health guru Gary Null in New York City has devoted several segments of his popular radio program extolling the benefits of the urine cure. Occasionally, it is mentioned or examined in magazines, newspapers, TV and in movies. There are over eighty websites reviewing different viewpoints on urine therapy and over a dozen books written on the subject, still, the majority of people are unaware of its value.

Acknowledgement of urine therapy in the West goes to the late Dr. John A. Armstrong, who was among the first to do pioneering research in this field. Armstrong's inspiration came from Proverbs 5:15 in the Old Testament which says: "Drink water out of thine own cisterns." He fasted on his own urine and water for forty-five days to heal himself from tuberculosis. He also used urine therapy to cure his diseased foot. He suffered a grave laceration to his toes, ankle and foot. He applied saturated old urine to the affected parts. The bandages were kept moist by repeated soakings but were not removed until the fifth day. When finally removed, the results were astonishing; all trace of the injury had disappeared, and the foot was healthy and supple as it had ever been. The whole medical world was thrown into turmoil when his book, *The Water of Life*, was published. His book documents numerous patients who had been snatched from the jaws of death through the efficacy and harmlessness of urine therapy. For years, he supervised many people on urine fasts, including terminal patients thought to be incurable. According to Armstrong, any disease could be treated with urine therapy including venereal diseases, cancer, leukemia, malaria, dropsy and gangrene. Extraordinarily, he treated everyone without diagnosis.

Another pioneer was Martha Christie, who wrote *Your Own Perfect Medicine*. She asserted that urine therapy helped her overcome several complications, including menstrual problems, pelvic inflammation, ulcerative colitis, Chron's disease, chronic fatigue syndrome, thyroid disorders and mononucleosis. In her book, she cites more than fifty research and clinical studies that detail urine's healing properties. Many of these are aged reports by doctors and medical scientists giving patients injections of their own urine. These case studies feature amazing results overcoming candida, colitis, cancer, diabetes, depression and a host of other health problems. Also included is a report how safe and effective urine was in treating external wounds during wartime. Her book is considered one of the most authoritative on the subject of urine therapy.

Here are some sample testimonies of people whose health has been restored:

- ✓ I had been suffering from migraines for twenty years. Because I also suffered from rheumatoid arthritis, I was often taking painkillers. Then I started drinking my urine. A few months later, my arthritis has disappeared, and so did my headaches.

- ✓ I had hay fever and allergies whenever the seasons changed. I tried the over-the-counter drugs, but they were expensive and didn't always help. So I took the advice of a friend and started urine therapy. In just two days of doing it, I was able to breathe more easily without the sniffles, the runny nose and eyes.

- ✓ I am a PWA (person with AIDS) and have been doing urine therapy for two and half months. My lymphadenopathy was gone within forty-eight hours after starting urine. I had a severe acne problem on my back. After five weeks, the skin was clear. My energy level increased enormously within a few days of drinking my urine.

- ✓ I am a paramedic worker at Bethany Colony where people with leprosy are treated. We achieved good results with this treatment. I have treated many cases and the treatment has never failed. The problem is that the patient is often unwilling to drink his or her own water. Therefore we mix it with some juice and serve it for breakfast. I can honestly say it is the best treatment for leprosy ulcers, asthma, and several skin disorders. I am extremely grateful for this therapy and plan to start a small clinic for urine therapy.

- ✓ A young woman had developed a growth in her breast. She was put on a diet of her own urine plus tap water and used urine compresses. In a short time, four days, the growth had entirely disappeared.

- ✓ After a number of weeks in which I ritually drank my own morning urine, I noticed that changes were slowly beginning to take place in my body. Now after using urine for fourteen years, I can confirm that I am 99 percent less susceptible to all kinds of epidemics, flu, infections, and other miseries I used to be very susceptible to. You do not have to be sick to start urine therapy. It increases your resistance to disease.

✓ In the last five years, I have gone through three serious operations. I had many difficult illnesses including arthritis, rheumatism, glaucoma, high blood pressure, a blood clot that cause my leg to turn black from the knee down due to no blood circulation, pancreatic problems that caused a swollen tongue and an inability to take food properly. After drinking my own water for seven months, all the toxins in my body disappeared. I visited the doctor for a check-up afterward. He was shocked and surprised saying I was completely normal. It is a wonderful medicine. Once you know this information, you won't need any pills, vitamins, or hormone shots. It is a gift from God.

✓ A young man, twenty-eight, was given three days to live. His condition was variously diagnosed as either cancer of the gullet or venereal disease. Through urine therapy the patient was completely cured.

✓ MQ contacted malaria and had it for three years. During the year before the treatment, he had suffered from thirty six attacks. He used to dose himself regularly with quinine. He finally cured himself completely with a urine fast lasting ten days.

✓ In Egypt, rescue workers found a thirty-seven-year-old man alive in earthquake rubble. He survived almost eighty-two hours by drinking his own urine. His wife, daughter, and mother would not and they died.

✓ Urine therapy healed and prevented a recurrent throat infection Joe had every few months for almost twenty years.

✓ Ms. P. suffered from rheumatism for years, especially in the hands. I started treating my hands with urine compresses daily. The result was extraordinary. Besides the fact that my hands felt much smoother, the most remarkable thing was that the pain practically disappeared

✓ L.V. had a fever of 104 degrees and was dehydrated two days in a row. She refused to go to the hospital because of previous bad experiences. She drank her own urine, within twenty minutes, she started sweating, and the fever started going down and down to 85 degrees. She slept for six hours. Upon awakening she had diarrhea and her temperature was normal.

✓ Diagnosed with metastatic cancer of the liver, complicated by hepatitis, she was sent home to die. She drank only her first morning urine and used it externally, no fasting. After ten days, she went back to the doctor feeling much better. The doctor could not believe she was alive. Within a few weeks she was working again.

✓ I was suffering from amoebic dysentery for the last twenty years and my physicians assured me it would accompany me forever. I was also having eczema since more than forty years. To my utter surprise, I got rid of both major diseases by using urine therapy.

✓ Andre K. suffered for years with arteriosclerosis. The circulation problems in his arms caused both numbness and pain. A few weeks after he started the recommended oral urine therapy in conjunction with massages, the pain ceased.

✓ Lisa L. had mosquito bites on her back and the urge to scratch was driving her crazy. She placed a urine soaked t-shirt on her back and after a half hour the itch disappeared.

✓ During the nine-day war in Jordan, the Red Crescent, the Islamic equivalent of the Red Cross, advised people against drinking polluted water by radio broadcasts, saying, "Your children are expiring of thirst, we cannot help you except by telling you that you may be able to save their lives by letting them drink their own urine."

✓ She has very dry skin to the extent that she gets deep cracks. They are very painful and do not heal easily. External use of urine therapy every two hours relieved the pain almost instantly and the cracks healed within twelve hours.

✓ I started to massage my face with fresh urine, and later with old urine. After two days, I noticed that the urine had an unusual effect on my skin. My pores, which were often oily, were much cleaner and the skin softer.

✓ I was in a motorcycle accident, breaking my arm in three places, scraping the skin on my shoulder, arm trunk, and leg. One side of my body was road burned several layers deep. I had no insurance so went home to heal myself. All I had for healing was my own urine. I applied it all over the open wounds. I never had a scab. My healing was from the inside out. The body filled in from the bone to the muscles, and finally pink smooth skin. The regeneration on my head and eyebrow cannot be noticed today. I was back at work within one month.

A single drop of urine, which is diluted in a homeopathic mixture, is enough to stimulate the development of antibodies against any malignant microorganisms taking advantage of a weak immune system. This is a great alternative for antibiotics and is very easy to prepare. It works equally well for infants, children, adults and the elderly. It is effective in dealing with many viral and bacterial problems such as:

✓ any type of fever or infection including appendicitis
✓ kidney or bladder infections
✓ gum sensitivity in adults and teething babies
✓ eye, ear, and tooth infections
✓ pimples, carbuncles, and cysts
✓ lupus, allergies, and skin rash

- ✓ stomach viruses, diarrhea, vomiting, colic pain, or intestinal gas
- ✓ tonsillitis, laryngitis, and sore throat
- ✓ tumors in the lymphatic glands and nodes
- ✓ swollen and painful abscesses, glands, and nodes
- ✓ breast lumps and tumors, including cancerous ones
- ✓ infections caused by antibiotic resistant bacteria

Successful results have been demonstrated by many cancer patients who recovered using urine therapy. Current studies of urine therapy with AIDS show promising results. Very few people know that their urine is a marker that can be used to detect the toxicity in their bodies, the quality of their diet, and the consequences of their lifestyle. Opportunistic diseases do not affect healthy people whose immune system is stable. Utilizing urine therapy is the best prevention for disease because it strengthens the immune system. If the body defense system is strong, there is little chance of sickness. If the body weakens and breaks down from imbalance of the vital body nutrients, urine therapy is the fastest way to solve it, especially since no diagnosis is necessary to utilize it.

CHAPTER 8

HISTORY OF URINE THERAPY

U rine therapy is the most original, primitive and simple form of homeopathy. In short, urine therapy has been around for a very long time. The medicinal use of urine dates back to the earliest civilizations. It is often referred to as the world's oldest medicine. Even the founder of Western medicine, Hippocrates wrote about his explorations with the healing properties of urine. It has been passed down by every generation but has somehow fallen into obscurity. The awareness of the benefits of urine therapy can come in very handy in case of a disaster. Stories have been told of individuals who were trapped without food and water but who lived by drinking their own urine. Ancient travelers in deserts and on the seas knew how to make use of urine when their stock of water was exhausted and thereby they could reach their destinations safely. Similarly, it has been described in the journals of sailors that passengers on ships were induced to take their own urine when their ships were lost during storms or the supply of drinking water diminished. As a result, they could avoid death until they reached shore. Whether it is from bad weather, being lost, trapped, shipwrecked, or just being unable to get help when needed, it has helped more than a few individuals survive difficult times.

Unsurprisingly the use of urine as a medicine can still be found in the medical traditions of ethnic tribes, which are still in close contact with nature. Eskimos still use urine as a medicine. In India, the Yogis and the great spiritual masters are well aware of the miracles of this "sacred" fluid. It was driven underground and mostly the tantrics and Yogis accepted it as the most sacred and effective remedy for the ailing. It has long been regarded in India as indispensable for the preservation of health. So much so that it has an extremely lengthy and involved history in India dating back over five thousand years. The use of urine is also rooted in the European tradition. Doctors in ancient Greece reportedly used urine for healing wounds. The Romans considered the medicinal use of urine in the treatment of wounds, dog and snake bites, skin diseases, eye infections, bruises and burns.

Urine therapy also has historical roots in ancient Egypt, Greece, Rome, the Aztec empire and since the Middle Ages in Europe. The history of drinking urine for therapeutic purposes dates back to the Holy Roman Empire when great urinal troths were erected in public squares of each city-state for residents to both contribute to, and benefit from. For hundreds of years, many European cultures including Russia have used urine to treat a wide variety of health problems. The ancient Indian text of Shivambu Kalpa Vidhi calls it the divine nectar that is capable of abolishing various types of diseases and ailments. Many religions have given importance to the drinking of urine. Many practitioners of the allopathic and ayurvedic systems have used it successfully in treating large numbers of patients. For centuries, European Gypsies have known about the curative powers of urine. In China, Mongolian priests and monks knew well and practiced the art of urine therapy. It has been reported that the Lamas of Tibet reach extended ages by drinking their own urine. For over five hundred years, Native Indians in the Western Hemisphere had knowledge of this remedy. So much so that indigenous people of Mexico, Argentina, Peru, and Chile continue to consume it for illnesses and utilize it as an antiseptic to treat wounds. In England, France, and probably elsewhere, the custom of washing one's hands in urine for its softening and beautifying properties still exists among the ladies. Urine has also been used even as a curative for animals and plants.

In the beginning of the eighteenth century, the dentists of Paris, France, used to apply urine for curing dental problems. The use of urine as a tooth wash is still found in many parts of Europe and America. Peasants in Portugal washed their clothes in urine, as did sailors out at sea. Irish, German, and Scandinavian women who have immigrated to the United States add human urine to the water to be used for cleansing clothing. In 1829, the physician Dioscorides advocated that the patient drink his own urine in cases of snake bites, poisons, bites of scorpions, mad dogs, etc. In the *Englishman's Treasure*, published in 1641, it gives a cure for wounds in which it is directed to wash the wounds very clean with urine. One's own urine was drunk as a preservative from the plague in early Europe. In the Civil War, the use of urine had been used as a remedy for scurvy. In South America, urine is still used as a common means of medicine. In New England, it was found to be a sure cure for jaundice. In the 19th century, the old people of central New York made lye tea from human urine and lime water to prevent colds. In olde Virginia and Maryland, it was known as a cure for eye problems and toothaches. Chemists in England have prepared the best types of bathing soaps and quality creams from it.

Throughout history, urine has played a part in the preparation and use of medicines produced on an alchemical basis. Human urine has been considered a healing agent in many Asian cultures for centuries. It has played an important role in the indigenous medical traditions all over the world. Ancient works on medicinal science have recorded their approval to the drinking of urine as a therapeutic measure. It has been an age-old tradition especially in sickness although many practice it for preventive health maintenance. Moreover, it had been kept a secret by healers and medicine men so they alone could have access to this "fountain of youth." It is no wonder that the ancient medicine men referred to it as "holy water".

In this day and age, The Water of Life Foundation in India and the Chinese Association of Urine Therapy promotes urine therapy for good health. It still plays an important role in some medical treatments in Germany, Japan, and has been gaining popularity in the United States. In Germany, urine treatments have been used since medieval times against all kinds of diseases. In Japan, urine therapy has been known for seven hundred years and is commonly prescribed even today against asthma, diabetes, and hypertension and on an experimental basis against AIDS and cancer.

The number of its uses is impressive and so are the numbers of its followers. According to Xinhua news agency more than three million Chinese drink urine to stay healthy. From India, in the state of Gujarat, there are nearly three hundred thousand users of urine therapy and in the city of Bombay nearly thirty-thousand plus are active users. Germany, Korea and Japan have a sizable number of citizens engaging in urine therapy. It is also growing in the West. In 2009, the Fifth World Congress Urotherapy was held in Guadalajara, Mexico, where advocates from around the world gathered to share their experiences. The 6th World Congress on Urotherapy is scheduled for Sydney, Australia, in 2013. In addition to naturopathic doctors, more and more allopathic doctors are attending these conferences to learn more about it. Today, numerous laboratories all over the world are engaged in research directed at the isolation of therapeutically valuable substances contained in human urine. It is even being utilized in the preparation of modern cosmetics and therapeutic drugs.

It is only a matter of time until it emerges as an accepted natural home remedy for people who want a fast, efficient and inexpensive way to improve their health.

CHAPTER 9

GETTING STARTED

The most convenient way to learn more about urine theapy is on the internet. Three good websites to learn about the history, science and approaches of this unique cure are:

- ✓ http://www.urinetherapeutics.com
- ✓ http://munot.in/about_urine_therapy
- ✓ http://www.all-natural.com/urine.html

Our bodies know what is going on inside them, and can diagnose problems before the physical symptoms are detected. That is why a urinalysis is done as a part of a routine medical exam. It is a very useful test in the diagnosis of and screening for many diseases and conditions. A complete urinalysis includes physical, chemical, and microscopic examinations. Urinalysis is invaluable because it goes deep into the cellular structures of the body. It alerts the physician to the presence of any disease. The secret to good health is to ingest these re-filtered components so the body's immune system can begin to make antibodies for the sickness. We should be very grateful to our kidneys. Not only do perform an impeccable diagnosis, they also produce a custom-made prescription for our own self-healing. If more people knew how to pay attention and listen to their body, they could stay healthy much longer.

Most people are surprised to learn that a baby in the mother's womb drinks their own urine in the form of amniotic fluid. This liquid is a critical contributor to the development of the fetus. Learning how the kidneys work to create urine will go a long way toward dispelling any concepts that urine is a waste product. The age-old concept prevailing in our society is that urine is poisonous or dirty excreta of the body. But his fallacy is proved wrongbased on successful research and experiments done with human urine. Another challenge is that urine is generally described as having an unpleasant odor. Their taste is considered so bad that the very idea of drinking it creates nausea. There is the concept of foul smell and disagreeable taste that needs to be dealt with. This difficulty is foremost in those who have never made an attempt to drink it. Some medicines and liquors are far more distasteful and have much more foul odors. Mixing it with water or juice greatly conceals the taste. In addition, eating vegetables and fruit will actually give it a favorable taste. In fact, once the pain of our physical problems becomes stronger than our concepts or fears, reception of urine therapy happens naturally. A good number of people will try it as a last resort to overcome their pain or sickness.

The only disadvantage of urine therapy is in acceptance, both by society as method of treatment, and by the individual who must drink it to be cured. The thought of drinking their urine may offend the sensibilities of some Westerners. This initial revulsion is usually based on concepts that are based on ignorance or fears. Social mores and customs are difficult to overcome so those who find it difficult to overcome negative feelings should begin by using it externally. The next time you have to go the bathroom, smell it and rub some on the back of your hand. The initial fear is the hardest, after that there is a natural learning curve to experiment with it. The easiest way to check it out is next time you get a scrape or a cut, apply some on a cotton ball and observe the results. When one sees the effect it has on the skin, they will begin to understand its efficacy. In fact, one of the great paradoxes of life is that not only is urine not poisonous but it is a universal panacea for any infection.

There are some simple ways to overcome the feelings of aversion of drinking your own water. Since the taste depends largely on diet and liquid intake, a vegetarian diet helps a great deal. Ultimately, the only way to know is to take the test, risk it and start. Forget all the thoughts that you have connected with urine since the beginning of our life. Start by touching your urine covered finger with your tongue. Once you make this leap of faith and you find out for yourself that it is not all that bad, it is easy and natural. Start with a few drops, taking a small amount then increase gradually. You can even make a homeopathic preparation from just a few drops. This mixture contains no taste or color.

The most common recommended dosage is 2 to 4 oz. of fresh urine once daily in the morning as a tonic for keeping healthy and as prevention against illnesses. A chaser of pure water after swallowing eliminates any taste of urine from lingering in the mouth. Mixing it with fruit juice or your favorite beverage is a great option. The first morning urine is the most efficacious against combating disease and maintaining optimum health. The rationale is that after the body has rested during the night, the accumulation of minerals, hormones, and vital elements contained in urine are in higher concentration, making the first morning urine the most potent elixir. Anyone who is in a diseased state is strongly encouraged to take an increased dosage. Any increase intake will be helpful toward a speedy recovery. There are no side effects no matter how much is ingested. You cannot overdose from it. It is 96 percent water along with the blood's filtered, vital components. Urine therapy is not recommended while on prescribed medications or recreational drugs. The methods and administering techniques can always be adjusted to personal preferences. Those who drink it regularly say the taste is mild and not unpleasant at all—a bit salty, like broth or seawater. The taste depends on your constitution and your daily diet. Everything you eat and drink has an effect on your urine. If you eat spicy or fast food, then you will recognize that it has a stronger or somewhat bitter taste. You will also notice that when you are sick the taste is more pungent than when you feel healthy – this is normal because your body is making the antibodies to correct its metabolism. Most people start to think seriously about what they eat once they start to drink their own water. A change in dietary habits plays an important role in the healing process.

After the initial re-introduction of the body's own medicine, be prepared as the healing process may begin. Remember that urine comprises the sum of all the experiences the body has had. Records of infections, allergies and diseases are stored within our urine. Depending on the toxicity, the body will begin to purify itself. In the detoxification period, poisonous substances that have been stored in the body for years are released. The body might start to fight certain viruses by increasing the temperature and causing a fever. During the healing crisis, symptoms such as a rash, sweating, fever, diarrhea, vomiting, headache or coughing may arise. General feebleness may be felt as a result of the excess toxins, and in such a case plenty of sleep, rest and good food will help. When we confront the immune system with this information for a second time, we stimulate the body's natural mechanisms for an effective defense. By stimulating the body's natural powers, real healing takes place. Urine contains antibodies and immune stimulating factors against all viruses, harmful bacteria and fungi. The self-inoculation of urine is similar to when a flu shot introduces a virus into the body to make antibodies for it. Afterwards, the majority feel much better in a few hours to a few days.

To restate again, urine therapy consists of two parts: internal application (e.g., drinking urine) and external application (e.g., massaging with urine). Both aspects are important and complement each other. The easiest way to start is by using it externally. Urine is skin food and will rebuild tissues. It has miraculous healing abilities in the treatment of painful and disabling wounds, cuts, sores, bites, stings, blisters and rashes especially the ones which refuse to heal. For skin problems such as gangrene, psoriasis, eczema and dermatitis, urine pack works well and can even prevent scar tissue. A urine compress should be moistened regularly and renewed several times daily. The use of old urine is suggested for wounds, rashes or other skin legions. Urine can be three to four days old and stored at regular room temperature so that fermentation can take place. Urine therapy offers complete recovery for serious burns instead of unsightly scars, tightly puckered skin and stiffened limbs. Armstrong insisted that cures were faster and more effective in those who massaged themselves with urine.

During any form of internal use of urine, the following should be observed:

- ✓ Urine therapy should not be started if medical or any other form of treatment is being used. Two days should intervene between the stopping of medication and the commencement of urine therapy.
- ✓ Diet for the most intense forms of the internal technique, should be low in protein and salt. Refined, processed, and synthetic foods should be avoided, for example, white sugar, refined flour, tinned food, and so on. Spicy food may make the urine pungent and difficult to drink. Some proponents recommend that milk consumption be stopped too.
- ✓ Intake of alcohol and tobacco should be reduced to the barest minimum, or preferably avoided totally if possible.

✓ A healing crisis is said to be a sign that the body is purifying itself very rapidly. These crises may take the form of loose stools, skin eruptions such as pimples and boils, vomiting, fever of unexplained origin, cough, general weakness and debility. If healing crises occur, the best way to handle the situation is to reduce the intake of urine or to stop completely and rest the body. Do not run to your doctor and start taking medications to suppress the healing crisis. Let them unfold naturally and according to their own sequences. The following are the most common manifestations of the healing crises and their recommended treatment:

✓ Loose stools—fasting and complete rest for one day is probably the best measure. Plenty of boiled or distilled water and lemon juice is suggested. The toxins of the body that have been loosened then have a chance to be eliminated.

✓ Skin eruptions such as pimples and boils can be treated in the following ways. In the early stages, rub the lesion with urine and leave the urine on for one or two hours before washing if off to stop the process. If they continue to cause trouble or if boils develop, urine packs can be applied.

✓ Vomiting may occur when the urine is especially bad tasting and smelling as in fevers, jaundice and other illnesses. The urine of such diseases may seem totally unpalatable, yet if the patient has steeled his mind to drink it, then copious supplies of water will help to dilute the urine and make it easier to drink. If you can hold down the first flow, then the second should be more dilute and better tasting, and so on, until clear pleasant tasting urine finally comes. Vomiting is good in that it cleans the stomach. Therefore, it should not cause any undue worry. After vomiting, the nausea is usually relieved and you feel better. If vomiting persists and dry retching occurs, you should seek professional help. After vomiting urine, you should rest and take some light fluids such as lemon water.

✓ Mild fever of unexplained origin can occur as a reaction of the body, designed to burn up the toxins. It is one of the most thorough way to detox and requires nothing more than complete rest and constant fluid intake. After the fever, fruit and a light diet should precede the commencement of urine therapy.

✓ Cough and cold may appear and indicate elimination of mucus from the lungs and respiratory passages. *Neti* using half water and half urine is good to relieve all discomfort and to help wash out mucus form the nasal passages and sinuses. The diet should exclude milk and milk products and all mucus-producing foods such as fats and excessive starch until the cold is finished.

✓ General weakness may be felt as a result of the excess toxins, and in such a case plenty of sleep, rest and good food will help.

✓ In some diseases, the urine becomes dense, pungent, and seemingly unpalatable. It is advised that you attempt to utilize this urine even though it may be difficult to do so. Dense and scanty urine may contain mineral salts and other body components of value. Wash it down with plenty of water.

Each person is different, so the results of a friend's experimentation may not apply to you. Age, constitution, physique, diet, and disease all lead on a different path to the same goal - that of good health. Be patient, it is the most natural remedy, - the results may astonish you.

CHAPTER 10

CONCLUSION

Pollution is everywhere, not just in our city centers and industrial areas. Toxic chemicals can be in remote places, on mountains and in the depths of the ocean. Environmental contaminants are often undetectable to the senses. We may be unable to see the pollution in the air, taste the pathogens and chemicals in the water, or smell the pesticides in the food, but they are there. We cannot imagine that our chemically engineered ingenuity is endangering our very survival. Blood samples taken from citizens across the globe have toxins including pesticides, flame retardants, stain repellants, rocket fuel residues, heavy metals and quite a few other chemical compounds. Although it is hard to believe, even newborn babies are contaminated from the mother's placenta.

The human population, including the wildlife, is now threatened because of our separation from nature. We are sacrificing the whole planet for our own gratification.

- ✓ Each year, we spray over a billion pounds of pesticides on our crops.
- ✓ We feed millions of pounds of antibiotics to our farm animals.
- ✓ We inject our cattle with cycle after cycle of growth hormone.
- ✓ We eat grains contaminated with mycotoxins.
- ✓ We dump billions of tons of toxic waste into our waste sites and rivers.
- ✓ We drink water that has been poisoned with chlorine and fluoride.
- ✓ We drink diet sodas contaminated with aspartame.

✓ We breathe air that has been polluted with chemtrails.
✓ We let our doctors destroy our bodies with x-rays.
✓ We smoke cigarettes and drink lots of alcohol.
✓ We eat junk food, fast food and processed food.
✓ We breathe invisible nuclear radioactive isotopes.
✓ We shower with water that has been contaminated.
✓ We are surrounded by toxic heavy metals in our environment.

The hazardous substances found in air, food, soil, water and consumer products are linked to premature death and long list of adverse health effects including: cancer, cardiovascular disease, asthma, developmental disorders, gastrointestinal illnesses, neurodegenerative diseases such as Alzheimers and Parkinsons, decreases in IQ, premature birth, birth defects, immune system suppression and reproductive problems. Of increasing concern are endocrine-disrupting chemicals also known as hormone disruptors and gender benders. The connection between environmental factors and adverse health outcomes is becoming stronger and more direct. Toxicologists and epidemiologists are trying to understand the adverse health effects of thousands of chemicals. We are so chemically burdened that we can barely begin to figure out how to reverse or remedy the situation.

Most people are consistently exposed to substances that are known to damage our DNA. Radiation, plastics, cigarette smoke, chemicals in soft drinks, pesticides and others have all been found to damage our DNA. It is unfortunate that when our DNA is damaged, we subject ourselves to numerous health problems. Our cells become suppressed in producing what our bodies need and our bodies become more convoluted in re-growing healthy cells. Worse, the effects of our chemical habits and lifestyles are passed to our children and possibly to later generations. Our DNA has the ability to repair itself given the right enzymes and proteins. For anyone that has the resources and time, there are viable, alternative therapies (e.g. http://www.cancure.org/home.htm). Most of these individual therapies will provide the amino acids, the enzymes, minerals or compounds to reverse DNA breakdown. However, only urine therapy has all these ingredients and more to reverse the problem of genetic mutation caused by toxins.

Modern medicine doesn't emphasize the importance of knowing natural remedies. Most consumers feel that the knowledge of the body is best left in the hands of doctors, however, their dubious record raises serious questions about their aptitude. Oddly enough, we are the best doctor for our sicknesses. Misdiagnoses, unnecessary or incompetent surgery, errors in medication and high hospital infection rates do not inspire confidence in the current medical system. Most hospitals have to rely on strong medical intervention to relieve symptoms from the medical errors that occur on a daily basis. The FDA is supposed to look after our health yet they approve drugs that turn out to be gravely dangerous to health. This is very strange considering they have harmful side effects, cost more and have less success than alternative medicines. Consequently, more people are turning away from conventional medicine.

The practice of using one's own urine as a medicine and immune system booster is undoubtedly the most ancient remedy on the planet. Some of the chronic diseases that it is effective against include: cancer, heart disease, kidney failure, asthma, anemia, urinary diseases, colds, candida, diabetes, digestive problems, allergies and jaundice. Other problems such as injuries, warts, psoriasis, lumps and bites are often cured in a few days of treatment. The list of diseases for which it is effective is long enough to consider it a miracle remedy.

Urine therapy could be the medicine of the future for billions of people without health care. The medical establishment should adjust their system so that alternative medicines, like urine therapy, can be integrated seamlessly. This simple adjustment alone could tremendously reduce health care costs. The extra advantages of no diagnosis, no side effects and no costs make it more than an option. Urine therapy offers each individual the power to deal with any health crises efficiently, effectively and economically.

Despite many incredible medical discoveries, millions are still suffering or even crippled by illnesses today. The conventional medical profession has dominated society so that alternative medicines like urine therapy are almost unknown. Not only has the medical community conditioned us to believe that drugs and surgery are all that is needed to restore lost health, but they have ignored the research on the efficacy of urine therapy. The extensive medical research already done on this natural medicine has not been disseminated to the general public. Many more studies should be started on the efficacy of urine therapy for the many debilitating illnesses facing people today. Every year thousands of operations are performed and millions of prescription drugs are dispensed as proof that modern medicine cannot cure disease but can only control it at best. Meanwhile, researchers sat in their laboratories and watched as simple urea from urine completely destroyed rabies and polio viruses, tuberculosis, typhoid, gonorrhea, dysentery bacteria and cancer cells. They watched as it saved the lives of cancer patients, cured and relieved asthma, eczema, whooping cough, diabetes, arthritis and a host of other illnesses. The general public was never told about such discoveries yet modern health epidemics grew for the reason that urine therapy, unlike surgery and drugs, cannot be patented and sold for huge profits.

Believing there is a natural medicine that is free and can heal most ailments seems totally ludicrous. Particularly if you add the fact that it has been around for thousands of years and works both externally and internally. Until its curative powers have been experienced personally, utilizing urine to combat sicknesses will continue to sound impossible. It might not be admired but there are people all over the world that are healthy as a result of drinking their urine daily. There are millions more that can benefit if only the word can get out. Their very lives depend on it. More importantly, the health of future generations requires a safe, inexpensive way to deal with health issues. Urine therapy is an empirical method and its effectiveness has been proven by innumerable clinical tests. And there are thousands of testimonies of patients who were seriously ill but who were miraculously healed to prove it.

Its advantages are almost too good to be true:

- ✓ It conveys to the organism all the vitamins required by it.
- ✓ It enables antigens and antibodies, eliminated by the kidneys, to act effectively on the organism.
- ✓ This treatment performs hormonal regulation.
- ✓ It is a germicide, anti-poison and a tonic.
- ✓ It contains powerful antiseptic and antitoxic properties.
- ✓ It invigorates the body and removes weaknesses.
- ✓ It is nutritive, digestive, and a laxative.
- ✓ It heals and dries up wounds and soothes burns.
- ✓ It protects and restores to health every organ in the body.
- ✓ It is equally useful to males and females of all age groups.
- ✓ Requires no need for a doctor for the diagnosis of the illness.
- ✓ It is an easy, inexpensive and self-dependent means to health.

Through the internet, more and more people around the world are learning about this free, natural medicine. Urine is the ideal tonic for the restoration of health. Urine contains antigens, enzymes, hormones and the body's own genetic code. It is both a deterrent and remedy for all illnesses. It even gives an aged person the vitality and vigor of a youth. In brief, the medical use of urine ought to have public recognition before any more widespread, crippling health problems devastate humanity. Most people simply cannot afford conventional or even alternative medical treatments. Their best solution is this free, God-given remedy. Though sometimes considered an unpleasant last resort, it continues to be the hidden panacea for today's illnesses.

BIBLIOGRAPHY

Armstrong J.W. *A Treatise on Urine Therapy, the Water of Life* (1974). Health Science Press.

Baker, Nena. *The Body Toxic* (2008). New York, New York: North Point Press.

Bartnett, Beatrice and Adelman, Margie. *The Miracles of Urine Therapy* (1987).

Blanc, Paul D. *How Everyday Products Make People Sick* (2009). Berkeley, CA: University of California Press.

Bollet, M. D. and Alfred Jay. *Plagues and Poxes* (2004). New York: Demos Medical Publishing.

Bollinger, Ty *Cancer, Step Outside the Box* (2010). Infinity 510 Partners.

Boyd, David R. *Dodging the Toxic Bullet* (2010). Vancouver, BC, Canada: Greystone Books.

Christy, Martha. *Your Own Perfect Medicine* (1994). Arizona: Wishland Publishing.

Colbert, Don. *Toxic Relief* (2001). Lake Mary, FL: Siloam Press.

Collman, James P. *Naturally Dangerous* (2001). Sausalito, CA: University Science Books.

Cook, Christopher D. *Diet for A Dead Planet* (2004). New York: The New Press.

Desai, Morarjii. *Miracles of Urine Therapy.* New Delhi, India: Pankaj Publications.

Fitzgerald, Randall. *The Hundred Year LIE* (2006). New York: Dutton.

Fradkin, Philip L. *Fallout, an American Nuclear Tragedy* (2004). Colorado: Johnson Printing Co.

Gibson, Rosemary and Singh, Janardan Prasad. *Wall of Silence: The Untold Story of the Medical Mistakes That Kill and Injure Millions of Americans* (2003). Washington DC: Lifeline Press.

Gillard, Authur. *Food-Borne Diseases* (2011). Farmington Hills, MI: Greenhaven Press.

Glasstone, Samuel. *The Effects of Nuclear Weapons* (1962). Washington DC: U.S. Government Printing Office.

Gould, Jay M. *Deadly Deceit, Low Level Radiation, High-level Cover Up* (1990). New York: Four Walls, Eight Windows Publishing.

Haugen, David M. *Health Care* (2008). Farmington Hills, MI: Greenhaven Press.

Junger, Alejandro. *CLEAN* (2009). New York: Harper One.

Michaels, David. *Doubt Is Their Product* (2008). New York, New York: Oxford University Press.

Lara, Martin. *Uropathy, the Most Powerful Holistic Medicine* (1999). New York: The Uropathy Press.

National Academies Press. *Exposure of the American Population to Radioactive Fallout from Nuclear Weapons Test* (2002). Washington DC.

Nauneet Publications Limited. *Auto-Urine Therapy.* Gujarat, India.

O'Quinn, John F. *Urine Therapy* (2006). Pomeroy, Washington: Life Science Institute.

Parks, Peggy J. *Health Care* (2009). San Diego, CA: Reference Point Press.

Patel, Raojibhai. *Manav Mootra -Auto-Urine Therapy* (1997). Gujarat, India.

Pauling, Linus. *No More War!* (1983). New York: Dodd, Mead and Company,

Peschek-Bohmer, Flora and Schreiber, Gisela. *Urine Therapy* (1997). Vermont: Healing Arts Press.

Reid, T. R. *The Healing of America* (2009). New York: Penguin Press.

Rotblat, Joseph. *Nuclear Radiation in Warfare* (1982). Oelgeschlager Gunn and Hain.

Schapiro, Mark. *Exposed: The Toxic Chemistry of Everyday Products and What's at Stake for American Power* (2007). White River Junction, Vermont: Chelsea Green Publishing.

Sharma, S. K. *Miracles of Urine Therapy* (2005). New Delhi, India: Diamond Books.

Shoemaker, Ritchie C. *Mold Warriors* (2005). Baltimore, MD: Otter Bay Books.

Smith, Rick and Lourie, Bruce. *Slow Death by Rubber Duck* (2009). Berkeley, CA: Counterpoint.

Somers, Suzanne. *Knockout* (2009). New York, New York: Three Rivers Press.

Sternglass, Ernest. *Secret Fallout* (1981). New York: McGraw-Hill Publishing.

Tamplin, Arthur R. and Gofman, John W. *Population Control through Nuclear Pollution* (1970). Chicago, Il: Nelson-Hall Co. Publishers.

Takkar, G. K. *Wonders of Uropathy—Urine Therapy as a Universal Cure* (1996).

New Delhi, India: B. Jain Pubishers,

Tietel, Martin. *Genetically Engineered Food, Changing the Nature of Nature* (2001). Rochester, Vermont: Park Street Press.

Tietze, Harald W. *Urine, the Holy Water* (1996). New Delhi, India: B. Jain Publishers,

Van der Kroon, Coen. *The Golden Fountain: The Complete Guide to Urine Therapy* (1993).

Wagner, Viqi. *Do Infectious Diseases Pose a Serious Threat?* (2005). Detroit Michigan: Greenhaven Press.

Weil, Andrew. *Why Our Health Matters* (2009). New York: Hudson Street Press.

———. *You Can't Afford to Get Sick* (2011). New York: The Penguin Group.

Williams, Mary E. *Epidemics* (2005). Detroit, MI: Greenhaven Press.

REFERENCES

Chapter 1

- ✓ UN: Deaths up from cancer, diabetes, heart disease - WTOP.com. 2011. Available at http://www.wtop.com/?nid=267&sid=2431107.
- ✓ List of infectious diseases - Wikipedia, the free encyclopedia. 2011. Available at http://en.wikipedia.org/wiki/List_of_infectious_diseases.
- ✓ Diseases and Conditions - MayoClinic.com. 2011. Available at http://www.mayoclinic.com/health/DiseasesIndex/DiseasesIndex.
- ✓ Asthma and Allergy Foundation of America - Information About Asthma, Allergies, Food Allergies and More! 2011. Available at http://www.aafa.org/display.cfm?id=9&sub=30.
- ✓ National Center for Complementary and Alternative Medicine [NCCAM] - nccam.nih.gov Home Page. 2011. Available at http://nccam.nih.gov/.
- ✓ Health Issues—Global Issues. Available at http://www.globalissues.org/issue/587/health-issues.

Chapter 2

- ✓ 12th Report on Carcinogens (RoC) - National Toxicology Program. 2011. Available at http://ntp-server.niehs.nih.gov/go/roc12.
- ✓ 2011 | Children's Environmental Health Network. 2011. Available at http://www.cehn.org/articles/ma/2011.
- ✓ 50 years later - EPA says Teflon may contain toxic chemical [Archive] - Online Debate Network. 2011. Available at http://www.onlinedebate.net/forums/archive/index.php/t-2283.html?s=f5d483f727e9b35e7a42ff26e6807080.

✓ A List of Toxins, Where They Are Found, And How I Can Protect Myself From Them. 2011. Available at http://www.immune-health-solutions-for-you.com/list-of-toxins.html.

✓ Air Pollution. 2011. Available at http://www.niehs.nih.gov/health/topics/exposure/air-pollution/index.cfm.

✓ AllGov - Department of Health and Human Services - National Toxicology Program. 2011. Available at http://www.allgov.com/Agency/National_Toxicology_Program.

✓ A–Z List of Substances | IRIS | US EPA. 2011. Available at http://cfpub.epa.gov/ncea/iris/index.cfm?fuseaction=iris.showSubstanceList.

✓ CDC - Chemical Weapons Elimination - Methods Used to Destroy Chemical Warfare Agents. 2011. Available at http://www.cdc.gov/nceh/demil/methods.htm.

✓ CDC - National Report on Human Exposure to Environmental Chemicals - NER. 2011. Available at http://www.cdc.gov/exposurereport/.

✓ CDC – Occupational Cancer – Carcinogen List – NIOSH Safety and Health Topic. 2011. Available at http://www.cdc.gov/niosh/topics/cancer/npotocca.html.

✓ Centers for Disease Control and Prevention. 2011. Available at http://www.cdc.gov/.

✓ Chemical Fact Sheets | Pollution Prevention and Toxics | US EPA. 2011. Available at http://www.epa.gov/chemfact/.

✓ Climate Change Forcing Buried Toxics Back Into Atmosphere, Scientists Say | SolveClimate News. 2011. Available at http://solveclimatenews.com/news/20110725/climate-change-scientists-persistent-organic-pollutants-pops-toxics-arctic.

✓ Collaborative on Health and the Environment: Welcome. 2011. Available at http://www.healthandenvironment.org/.

✓ Harmful Chemicals in our Environment. 2011. Available at http://www.planetagenda.com/chemicals.htm.

References

- ✓ Health Services Research & Public Health Information Programs. 2011. Available at http://www.nlm.nih.gov/hsrph.html.
- ✓ Home - EcoHealth Alliance - Formerly Known as Wildlife Trust. 2011. Available at http://www.ecohealthalliance.org/.
- ✓ FDA says studies on triclosan, used in sanitizers and soaps, raise concerns. 2011. Available at http://www.washingtonpost.com/wp-dyn/content/article/2010/04/07/AR2010040704621.html.
- ✓ Federal and State Regulatory Agencies - Links - Integrated Environmental Management, Inc. 2011. Available at http://www.iem-inc.com/linkreg.html.
- ✓ Environmental Health News: Front Page. 2011. Available at http://www.environmentalhealthnews.org/.
- ✓ Environmental Health Perspectives: Monthly Journal of Peer-Reviewed Research and News on the Impact of the Environment on Human Health. 2011. Available at http://ehp03.niehs.nih.gov/home.action.
- ✓ Home - National Toxicology Program. 2011. Available at http://ntp-server.niehs.nih.gov/.
- ✓ Pesticide Action Network. 2011. Available at http://www.panna.org/. Report on Carcinogens (RoC) - National Toxicology Program. 2011. Available at http://ntp.niehs.nih.gov/index.cfm?objectid=72016262-BDB7-CEBA-FA60E922B18C2540.
- ✓ Safe Detoxification for Heavy Metal Poisoning. 2011. Available at http://www.evenbetterhealth.com/heavy-metal-poisoning.php#.TnUK397iI9Q.email.
- ✓ Science-Based Medicine Recycle. 2011. Available at http://www.sciencebasedmedicine.org/index.php/recycle/.
- ✓ Known and Probable Human Carcinogens. 2011. Available at http://www.cancer.org/Cancer/CancerCauses/OtherCarcinogens/GeneralInformationaboutCarcinogens/known-and-probable-human-carcinogens.

✓ WHO | Ten chemicals of major public health concern. 2011. Available at http://www.who.int/ipcs/assessment/public_health/chemicals_phc/en/index.html.

✓ Showering or bathing in chlorinated tap water—danger. 2011. Available at http://www.bidness.com/esd/showering.htm.

✓ Girls Exposed in Womb to BPA Have Risk of Behavior Problems - Bloomberg. Available at http://www.bloomberg.com/news/2011-10-24/girls-exposed-in-womb-to-bpa-have-risk-of-behavior-problems.html.

✓ How Chinese Babies Pay the Price for Chinese Pollution - Ecocentric - TIME Available at http://ecocentric.blogs.time.com/2011/10/19/how-chinese-babies-pay-the-price-for-chinese-pollution/.

✓ Campaign for Safe Cosmetics : Index. Available at http://www.safecosmetics.org/.

✓ Secret "Watch List" Reveals Failure To Curb Toxic Air: NPR. Available at http://www.npr.org/2011/11/07/142035420/secret-watch-list-reveals-failure-to-curb-toxic-air.

✓ Toxicokinetics. Available at http://www.eoearth.org/article/Toxicokinetics.

✓ Pollution Prevention Act of 1990 | Pollution Prevention | EPA. at http://www.epa.gov/p2/pubs/p2policy/act1990.htm

✓ Senator Frank R. Lautenberg.(Safe Chemicals Act) at http://lautenberg.senate.gov/newsroom/record.cfm?id=323863

✓ Toxics Release Inventory (TRI) Program | US EPA. at http://www.epa.gov/tri/

✓ Mercury and Air Toxics Standards | US Environmental Protection Agency. at http://www.epa.gov/mats/

Chapter 3

✓ CDC - 2011 Estimates of Foodborne Illness. 2011. Available at http://www.cdc.gov/foodborneburden/2011-foodborne-estimates.html.

✓ CDC and ADA Now Advise to Avoid Using Fluoride. 2011. Available at http://articles.mercola.com/sites/articles/archive/2010/11/13/cdc-and-ada-now-advise-to-avoid-using-fluoride.aspx.

✓ CDC Media Relations - Press Release on Diabetes Increase: 2011 .Available at http://www.cdc.gov/media/pressrel/2010/r101022.html.

✓ Chemicals In Our Waters Are Affecting Humans And Aquatic Life In Unanticipated Ways. 2011. Available at http://www.sciencedaily.com/releases/2008/02/080216095740.htm.

✓ Food Additives ~ CSPI's Food Safety. 2011. Available at http://www.cspinet.org/reports/chemcuisine.htm.

✓ Food Contaminants & Adulteration. 2011. Available at http://www.fda.gov/Food/FoodSafety/FoodContaminantsAdulteration/default.htm.

✓ HEALTH EFFECTS OF CHLORINE IN DRINKING WATER. 2011. Available at http://www.pure-earth.com/chlorine.html.

✓ Toxins in Food, Vaccines, Air, Water, and The Environment. 2011. Available at http://www.sssalas.com/ToxicEnviroments.html.

✓ The Invisible Toxic Drug That's Lurking in Your Water Supply. 2011. Available at http://articles.mercola.com/sites/articles/archive/2011/08/07/professional-perspectives-documentary.aspx?e_cid=20110807_SNL_Art_1.

✓ Fluoride Action Network. 2011. Available at http://www.fluoridealert.org/.

✓ CDC FoodNet. 2011. Available at http://www.cdc.gov/foodnet/.

✓ List of the Widely Known Dangerous Ingredients-Body and Food Products. Available at http://www.purezing.com/living/toxins/living_toxins_dangerousingredients.html.

Chapter 4

- ✓ An Introduction to CRCPD. Available at http://www.crcpd. org/about/about.aspx.
- ✓ IEER Press Release: Nuclear Testing Fallout Attributed to Cancers, U.S. Government Study Shows. Available at http:// www.ieer.org/comments/fallout/pr0202.html.
- ✓ History of Nuclear Weapons Testing. Available at http:// archive.greenpeace.org/comms/nukes/ctbt/read9.html.
- ✓ The Nuclear Weapon Archive - A Guide to Nuclear Weapons. Available at http://www.nuclearweaponarchive.org/.
- ✓ Radioactive I-131 from Fallout - National Cancer Institute. Available at http://www.cancer.gov/cancertopics/causes/i131.
- ✓ 9 Everyday Sources of Radiation - 1 - MSN Health - Cancer Slide Show. 2011. Available at http://health.msn.com/health-topics/cancer/9-everyday-sources-of-radiation.
- ✓ Higher cancer risk continues after Chernobyl - National Cancer Institute. Available at http://www.cancer.gov/ newscenter/pressreleases/2011/ChernobylRadiation.
- ✓ Iodine-131 detected in Nebraska, North Carolina, and Glasgow Truth Frequency News. Available at http:// truthfrequencynews.com/?p=1439. A
- ✓ All Levels of Radiation Confirmed to Cause Cancer. 2011. Available at http://www.commondreams.org/ news2005/0630-06.htm.
- ✓ Dangers of Electromagnetic Radiation. 2011. Available at http:// www.shareguide.com/radiation.html. Accessed August 5, 2011.
- ✓ ATSDR - Toxic Substances - Ionizing Radiation. 2011. Available at http://www.atsdr.cdc.gov/substances/ toxsubstance.asp?toxid=86.
- ✓ Electro Magnetic Field (EMF) - Hazardous to Our Health? 2011. Available at http://emf.mercola.com/sites/emf/emf-dangers.aspx.

✓ Environment: They Lied to Us - TIME. 2011. Available at http://www.time.com/time/magazine/article/0,9171,968800,00.html.

✓ CDC - EMF (Electric and Magnetic Fields) - NIOSH Workplace Safety and Health Topic. 2011. Available at http://www.cdc.gov/niosh/topics/emf/#emfpub.

✓ Fallout from Nuclear Weapons Tests and Cancer Risks *American Scientist*. 2011. Available at http://www.americanscientist.org/issues/feature/2006/1/fallout-from-nuclear-weapons-tests-and-cancer-risks.

✓ The Nuclear Scandal. *Time Magazine*. 1988. Available at http://www.time.com/time/magazine/article/0,9171,968800,00.html.

✓ The Radiation Effects Research Foundation Website. 2011. Available at http://www.rerf.jp/index_ea.html.

✓ Neutron radiation - Wikipedia, the free encyclopedia. 2011. Available at http://en.wikipedia.org/wiki/Neutron_radiation.

✓ Public Health Focus > Radiation Safety. 2011. Available at http://www.fda.gov/NewsEvents/PublicHealthFocus/ucm247403.htm.

✓ Radiation Information Network. 2011. Available at http://www.physics.isu.edu/radinf/.

✓ Radiation Nation - MSN Health - Cancer. 2011. Available at http://health.msn.com/health-topics/cancer/articlepage.aspx?cp-documentid=100271966&GT1=31025.

✓ Radiation Studies: Feasibility Study of Weapons Test Fallout | CDC RSB. 2011. Available at http://www.cdc.gov/nceh/radiation/fallout/default.htm.

✓ Radionuclides > FDA/ORA CPG 7119.14. 2011. Available at http://www.fda.gov/Food/FoodSafety/FoodContaminantsAdulteration/ChemicalContaminants/Radionuclides/ucm078331.htm.

✓ Report No. 160 - Ionizing Radiation Exposure of the Population of the United States (2009). 2011. Available at http://www.ncrppublications.org/Reports/160.

✓ Nuclear fallout - Wikipedia, the free encyclopedia. 2011. Available at http://en.wikipedia.org/wiki/Nuclear_fallout.

✓ Nuclear power plant accidents: listed, visualised and ranked since 1952 | World news | guardian.co.uk. 2011. Available at http://www.guardian.co.uk/news/datablog/2011/mar/14/nuclear-power-plant-accidents-list-rank.

✓ Nuclear power plants, world-wide. 2011. Available at http://www.euronuclear.org/info/encyclopedia/n/nuclear-power-plant-world-wide.htm.

✓ National Council on Radiation Protection & Measurements (NCRP) - Radiation Exposure Data, Radiation Protection Guidelines. 2011. Available at http://www.ncrponline.org/.

✓ List of civilian nuclear accidents - Wikipedia, the free encyclopedia. 2011. Available at http://en.wikipedia.org/wiki/List_of_civilian_nuclear_accidents#Scope_of_this_article.

✓ Health Effects | Radiation Protection | US EPA. 2011. Available at http://www.epa.gov/radiation/understand/health_effects.html. A

✓ Neutron radiation. 2011. Available at http://www.hps.org/publicinformation/ate/q609.html.

✓ List of military nuclear accidents - Wikipedia, the free encyclopedia. 2011. Available at http://en.wikipedia.org/wiki/List_of_military_nuclear_accidents.

✓ List of nuclear reactors - Wikipedia, the free encyclopedia. 2011. Available at http://en.wikipedia.org/wiki/List_of_nuclear_reactors.

✓ List of the More Widely Known Dangerous Ingredients in Body & Food Products. 2011.

✓ Infectious diseases are spreading more rapidly than ever before, WHO warns. Available at http://www.ncbi.nlm.nih.gov/pmc/articles/PMC1962876/.

✓ The Dangers of Nuclear Power: An Open Letter to Physicists. Available at http://www.ccnr.org/open_letter.html.

✓ Environmental impact of nuclear power - Wikipedia, the free encyclopedia. at <http://en.wikipedia.org/wiki/Environmental_impact_of_nuclear_power>

Chapter 5

✓ 195,000 People Die Every Year Due To Medical Malpractice. 2011. Available at http://www.godlikeproductions.com/forum1/message779999/pg1.

✓ New Study Finds Medical Error Rates are Underreported | The Rundown News Blog | PBS NewsHour | PBS. 2011. Available at http://www.pbs.org/newshour/rundown/2011/04/new-study-finds-medical-error-rates-are-underreported.html.

✓ Government Study Shows 15,000 Medicare Patients Die Each Month From Hospital Care | Nutrition And Diet News. 2011. Available at http://nutritiondietnews.com/government-study-shows-15000-medicare-patients-die-each-month-from-hospital-care/852345/.

✓ Medical Errors and Malpractice Stories. Available at http://www.squidoo.com/medicalerrors.

✓ Medical Malpractice Facts | eHow.com. 2011. Available at http://www.ehow.com/about_5389477_medical-malpractice.html.

✓ Medical Errors - A leading cause of Death. Available at http://www.cancure.org/medical_errors.htm.

✓ Insider's Guide: Avoid Getting Sick in the Hospital | HealthAngle. Available at http://www.healthangle.com/resources/avoid-hospital-sickness.

✓ New Alert System Aims to Reduce Deadly Medication Mistakes - WSJ.com. Available at http://online.wsj.com/article/SB10001424052748703626604575010932945077528.html.

✓ Study Puts Cost of Medical Errors At $19.5 Billion - Health Blog - WSJ. Available at http://blogs.wsj.com/ health/2010/08/09/study-puts-cost-of-medical-errors-at-195-billion/.

✓ What You Need to Know About Sepsis. Available at http:// knowledgebase.findlaw.com/kb/2010/Nov/208511.html.

✓ Methicillin-resistant Staphylococcus aureus - Wikipedia, the free encyclopedia. Available at http://en.wikipedia.org/wiki/ Mrsa.

✓ MRSA Risks & How To Prevent Staph Infection -- Natural Health Newsletter. Available at http://www.jonbarron. org/immunity/mrsa-methicillin-resistant-staphylococcus-staph.

✓ Press Release - Government Study Finds Lack of Progress in Preventing Medical Errors. Available at http://www.24-7pressrelease.com/press-release/government-study-finds-lack-of-progress-in-preventing-medical-errors-197628. php.

✓ Medical Malpractice Statistics. Available at http://www.2keller. com/library/medical-malpractice-statistics.cfm.

✓ Medical Malpractice Facts & Statistics on Hosptial Mistakes, Costs of Medical Malpractice Insurance. Available at http://www.resource4medicalmalpractice.com/topics/ medicalmalpracticefacts.html.

✓ A leading cause of Death. Available at http://www.cancure. org/medical_errors.htm.

✓ Prescription Painkiller Overdoses in the U.S. Available at http:// www.cdc.gov/Features/VitalSigns/PainkillerOverdoses/.

✓

Chapter 6

✓ Alternative Medicine:Self Urine Therapy - Shivambu By Munot.in - Introduction. 2011. Available at http://munot.in/ about_urine_therapy/introduction.

✓ DNA in Urine Can Reveal Disease | LiveScience. 2011. Available at http://www.livescience.com/977-dna-urine-reveal-disease.html.

✓ DNA Repair. 2011. Available at http://users.rcn.com/jkimball.ma.ultranet/BiologyPages/D/DNArepair.html.

✓ Drink Your Own Urine as Cocktail of The Day; Healthy Urine Therapy That Cures any Disease | Healthmad. 2011. Available at http://healthmad.com/alternative/drink-your-own-urine-as-cocktail-of-the-day-healthy-urine-therapy-that-cures-any-disease/.

✓ Is it Safe to Drink Your Urine? 2011. Available at http://www.buzzle.com/articles/is-it-safe-to-drink-your-urine.html.

✓ Is Urine Medicine? | Paxherbal Magazine. 2011. Available at http://paxherbalmagazine.com/paxmag/issue-18/urine.html.

✓ Microbial evaluation and public health implications of urine as alternative therapy in clinical pediatric cases: health implication of urine therapy. 2011. Available at http://www.ncbi.nlm.nih.gov/pmc/articles/PMC3032614/?tool=pmcentrez.

✓ Mutation, DNA Repair, and DNA Integrity | Learn Science at Scitable. 2011. Available at http://www.nature.com/scitable/topicpage/dna-damage-repair-mechanisms-for-maintaining-dna-344.

✓ New Vision Online: Urine: The wonder waste. 2011. Available at http://www.newvision.co.ug/D/9/34/765990.

✓ New way to study how enzymes repair DNA damage. 2011. Available at http://www.sciencedaily.com/releases/2010/01/100128165129.htm.

✓ Therapy: "Drink A glass of Urine" daily | The Health And Life Style. 2011. Available at http://www.sukiba.com/2011/07/therapy-drink-a-glass-of-urine-daily.html.

✓ Understand DNA Damage and Repair. 2011. Available at http://www.naturalnews.com/028736_DNA_damage_repair.html.

✓ Urine Contains Sex Hormones | Paxherbal Magazine. 2011. Available at http://paxherbalmagazine.com/paxmag/issue-18/hormones.html.

✓ Urine Is Blood | Paxherbal Magazine. 2011. Available at http://paxherbalmagazine.com/paxmag/issue-18/urine-blood.html.

✓ Urine Is Holistic Medicine | Paxherbal Magazine. 2011. Available at http://paxherbalmagazine.com/paxmag/issue-18/urine-is-holistic.html.

✓ Urine Is Life | Paxherbal Magazine. 2011. Available at http://paxherbalmagazine.com/paxmag/issue-18/life.html.

✓ Urine Is Natural Medicine | Paxherbal Magazine. 2011. Available at http://paxherbalmagazine.com/paxmag/issue-18/urine-natural.html.

✓ Urine therapy - MOM's Organic Market. 2011. Available at http://momsorganicmarket.com/ns/DisplayMonograph.asp?storeID=A6B40AE98C7842A98FC8DE4784880288&DocID=urinetherapy.

✓ Urine Therapy - The advantages of taking the piss - Drinking Your Own Urine. 2011. Available at http://www.fruitnut.net/HTML/201_Article_Urine.htm.

✓ Urine therapy - *The Freeman*: *The Freeman Sections Cebu Lifestyle*. 2011. Available at http://www.philstar.com/Article.aspx?articleId=728774&publicationSubCategoryId=111.

✓ Urine Therapy | Alternative Medicine Source. 2011. Available at http://alternativemedicinesource.com/urine-therapy/.

✓ Urine Therapy | Whole Health Chicago. 2011. Available at http://www.wholehealthchicago.com/363/urine-therapy/.

✓ Urine Therapy Benefits. 2011. Available at http://www.buzzle.com/articles/urine-therapy-benefits.html.

✓ Urine Therapy | Alternative Medicine Source. 2011. Available at http://alternativemedicinesource.com/urine-therapy/.

References

✓ Urine Therapy - The advantages of taking the piss - Drinking Your Own Urine. 2011. Available at http://www.fruitnut.net/HTML/201_Article_Urine.htm.

✓ Urine therapy - *The Freeman. The Freeman Sections Cebu Lifestyle*. 2011. Available at http://www.philstar.com/Article.aspx?articleId=728774&publicationSubCategoryId=111.

✓ Urine Therapy | Alternative Medicine Source. 2011. Available at http://alternativemedicinesource.com/urine-therapy/.

✓ Urine Therapy | Whole Health Chicago. 2011. Available at http://www.wholehealthchicago.com/363/urine-therapy/.

✓ Urine Therapy Benefits. 2011. Available at http://www.buzzle.com/articles/urine-therapy-benefits.html.

✓ Urine therapy for eczema. *The Real Supermum*. 2011. Available at http://www.therealsupermumblog.com/2011/07/19/urine-therapy-eczema/.

✓ Urine Therapy One Natural Solution To Plethora Of Diseases - Health Benefits Of Urine Therapy | Natural Remedies and Herbal Supplements. 2011. Available at http://www.greenherbalremedies.com/blog/urine-therapy-one-natural-solution-to-plethora-of-diseases/.

✓ Urine Therapy Shivambu. 2011. Available at http://www.scribd.com/doc/29352641/Urine-Therapy-Shivambu.

✓ Urine Therapy Works When Taken Judiciously | Paxherbal Magazine. 2011. Available at http://paxherbalmagazine.com/paxmag/issue-18/urine-therapy.html.

✓ Urine Therapy. A cure for all illnesses? 2011. Available at http://www.submityourarticle.com/articles/Patrick-Hamouy-2187/urine-therapy-17781.php.

✓ Urine Therapy: Is it Safe and Does it Work? 2011. Available at http://theyogadr.com/urine-therapy/.

✓ Urotherapy – A Treatment By making use of Urine | colitis treatment. 2011. Available at http://www.hangyukamengvip.com/urotherapy-a-treatment-by-making-use-of-urine/.

✓ Vitality Plus Australia. 2011. Available at http://tribreath.com.au/news/Urine-therapy---Traditional-Use-in-East--West-_368.htm.

✓ Antineoplastons (PDQ®) - National Cancer Institute. 2011. Available at http://www.cancer.gov/cancertopics/pdq/cam/antineoplastons/patient/page2.

✓ What is Urine therapy Therapy, Urine therapy Health Benefits, Definition. 2011. Available at http://naturalspedia.com/therapies/urine-therapy/whatistherapyhealthbenefitsdefinition.htm.

✓ WHO | Health topics. 2011. Available at http://www.who.int/topics/en/.

✓ WHO | World Health Organization. 2011. Available at http://www.who.int/csr/en/.

✓ YouTube - ⬚How Kidneys Work⬚. 2011. Available at http://www.youtube.com/watch?v=TzwPmz5V6Xg&feature=related.

✓ YouTube - ⬚Reabsorption in the Nephron⬚. 2011. Available at http://www.youtube.com/watch?v=KINOArtDeWg&feature=related.

✓ YouTube - ⬚The Urinary System⬚. 2011. Available at http://www.youtube.com/watch?v=chhNaLi9P3E.

✓ YouTube - ⬚Urinary system - The nephron⬚. 2011. Available at http://www.youtube.com/watch?v=aQZaNXNroVY&feature=player_embedded. Accessed July 4, 2011.

✓ YouTube - ⬚Urinary System | Anatomy | Biology⬚.2011. Available at http://www.youtube.com/watch?v=qxb2_d9ilEw&NR=1&feature=fvwp.

✓ YouTube - ⬚Urine therapy (your in good health)⬚. 2011. Available at http://www.youtube.com/watch?v=vrRhf3vNLLU.

References

✓ Urine Therapy for Cancer | eHow.com. 2011. Available at http://www.ehow.com/about_5432112_urine-therapy-cancer.html#ixzz1RvXPNqPL.

✓ Natural treatments for graves disease - Health Consultation | Provide health, fitness, science diet, psychological counseling, gender health, health products, disease prevention and other comprehensive information about. 2011. Available at http://www.health-consultation.com/natural-treatments-graves-disease/.

✓ Urine therapy. Available at http://www.vanderbilt.edu/AnS/psychology/health_psychology/Urine_Therapy.htm.

✓ Urine Therapy - Omaha's Heartland Healing Center. Available at http://www.heartlandhealing.com/pages/archive/urine_therapy/index.html.

✓ Urine Therapy: A cure for all diseases. Available at http://www.shirleys-wellness-cafe.com/urine.htm.

✓ Your Own Perfect Medicine? - Natural Health and Longevity Resource Center. Available at http://www.all-natural.com/urine.html.

✓ Complete Guide Urine Therapy. Available at http://universal-tao.com/article/urine_therapy.html.

✓ Urine Therapy Testimonials. Available at http://www.earthtym.net/ref-UT-notes-1.htm.

✓ Urine & Urea Therapy. Available at http://cancerresourcecenter.com/articles/alt114.html.

✓ Urine Therapy. Available at http://www.biomedx.com/urine/.

✓ Urine Therapy Community. Available at http://www.urine-therapy.org/.

✓ URINE & UREA Therapy. Available at http://www.health-science-spirit.com/urine.html.

✓ Wonders Of Urine Therapy. Available at http://www.lifepositive.com/Body/traditional-therapies/urine-therapy.asp.

- ✓ urine therapy/uropathy/breast cancer/ovarian cancer/ colon cancer/acid reflux/colic pain/colicky child/bloating/ indigestion/asthma/pneumonia/congestive heart failure/ parkinson/emphysema/ eczema/psoriasis/cystitis/kidney stones/fibroid tumor/cysts/eye infec. Available at http:// users.erols.com/martinlara/.
- ✓ P HELPS. Available at http://net-prophet.net/health/phelps/ phelps.htm.
- ✓ Urine. Available at http://www.goodmanlivingwell.com/ urine.htm.
- ✓ Urindya - Urine Therapy. Available at http://urindya.com/.
- ✓ Urotherapy - Exploration into Urine Therapy. Available at http://urotherapy.com/.
- ✓ Indian SANSKRIT DAMAR TANTRA SUTRA (part 5). Available at http://www.hps-online.com/hindiasutra.htm.
- ✓ Urine therapy - Wikipedia, the free encyclopedia. Available at http://en.wikipedia.org/wiki/Urine_therapy.
- ✓ Urophagia - Wikipedia, the free encyclopedia. Available at http://en.wikipedia.org/wiki/Urophagia.
- ✓ Urotherapy. Available at http://www.cancer. org/Treatment/TreatmentsandSideEffects/ ComplementaryandAlternativeMedicine/ PharmacologicalandBiologicalTreatment/urotherapy.
- ✓ UROTHERAPY FOR PATIENTS WITH CANCER. Available at http://www.indiadivine.org/audarya/ayurveda-health-wellbeing/932508-urotherapy-patients-cancer.html.
- ✓ Urine Therapy - The advantages of taking the piss - Drinking Your Own Urine. Available at http://www.fruitnut.net/ HTML/201_Article_Urine.htm.
- ✓ 5th World Congress Urotherapy. Available at http:// paraisodelasalud.org/5ocongreso/infocientifica_en.html.
- ✓ Urinary System Diagram. Available at http://www. medicalartlibrary.com/urinary-system-diagram.html.

- ✓ Urine therapeutics - information on urine therapy. Available at http://www.urinetherapeutics.com/index.htm.
- ✓ Urotherapy - Exploration into Urine Therapy. Available at http://urotherapy.com/.
- ✓ Urine Therapy: A cure for all diseases. Available at http://www.rexresearch.com/articles/urine.htm.
- ✓ Urotherapy. Available at http://www.cancer.org/Treatment/TreatmentsandSideEffects/ComplementaryandAlternativeMedicine/PharmacologicalandBiologicalTreatment/urotherapy.
- ✓ Urine: The body's own health drink? - Health News, Health & Families - The Independent. Available at http://www.independent.co.uk/life-style/health-and-families/health-news/urine-the-bodys-own-health-drink-467303.html.
- ✓ Urine Therapy/ Amaroli. Available at http://yoga.omgyan.com/cure/Urine-Therapy.html.
- ✓ Urine Therapy: The Science Of Drinking Your Own Pee - YouTube. Available at http://www.youtube.com/playlist?list=PL82C7822F6FCF0E3A.
- ✓ What Are the Uses of Urine Therapy for Cancer? Available at http://www.wisegeek.com/what-are-the-uses-of-urine-therapy-for-cancer.htm.

Chapter 7

- ✓ Urine Therapy: testimonials of cures. Available at http://www.shirleys-wellness-cafe.com/urine_testimonials.htm.
- ✓ Urindya - Urine Therapy. Available at http://www.urindya.com/intro.htm.
- ✓ Alternative Medicine:Self Urine Therapy - Shivambu By Munot.in http://munot.in/information_about_urine_therapy/self_experiences__case_history
- ✓ Urotherapy for patients with cancer. Available at http://www.csen.com/theory/cancer.htm.

Chapter 8
- ✓ Urine therapy - Wikipedia, the free encyclopedia. Available at http://en.wikipedia.org/wiki/Urine_therapy.

Chapter 9
- ✓ HPS Urine Therapy UT Programs. Available at http://www. hps-online.com/hurine4.htm.
- ✓ Choice of Therapy. Available at http://www.cancure.org/ choiceoftherapy.htm.

Made in the USA
San Bernardino, CA
30 August 2013